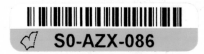

The Alzheimer's Sourcebook
for Caregivers

....

The Alzheimer's Sourcebook for Caregivers

A PRACTICAL GUIDE
FOR GETTING THROUGH THE DAY

UPDATED EDITION

Frena Gray-Davidson

LOWELL HOUSE
Los Angeles
CONTEMPORARY BOOKS
Chicago

Library of Congress Cataloging-in-Publication Data
Gray-Davidson, Frena
    The Alzheimer's Sourcebook for Caregivers: a practical guide for getting through the day/Frena Gray-Davidson
      p. cm.
    Includes bibliographical references and index.
    ISBN 1-56565-483-8 (second edition)
    1. Alzheimer's disease—Patients—Home care. 2. Alzheimer's disease—Patients—Family relationships. 3. Caregivers—Psychology. 4. Caregivers—Family relationships. I. Title
RC523.2.856 1993
362.1'96831—dc20
93-6363
CIP

Requests for such permissions should be addressed to:
Lowell House
2029 Century Park East, Suite 3290
Los Angeles, CA 90067

Publisher: Jack Artenstein
Associate Publisher, Lowell House Adult: Bud Sperry
Text Design: Tanya Maiboroda

Manufactured in the United States of America
10 9 8 7 6 5 4 3 2 1

Contents

Dedication

....

I had three remarkable teachers who opened my eyes to the Alzheimer's journey: Hilde Barglow, Sheila Moon, and Janet Weinstein.
Three courageous women.

I have two remarkable friends who have supported my own journey and I feel blessed by their presence in my life:

Janet B. Stern, life master extraordinaire, enthusiast, actress, and only incidentally octogenarian (but that will be our secret, Janet).

Barbara Sinton Wilson, cheerleader, supporter, friend, ally, role model, and wonderful human being.

Thank you, dear friends.

Foreword

When I first met Frena Gray-Davidson, she was part of a care-givers' group formed to care for an elderly woman in Berkeley, California, nearly a decade ago. Over the years, Frena has utilized her experience as a caregiver as well as her journalistic talent to gather information about how caregiving affects those who receive care, and also how it affects those who give it. She has acquired a great deal of practical knowledge about the business of daily living with a person severely impaired by Alzheimer's disease and has applied her creative insight to the problems inherent in that business. The result is a remarkably innovative and far-reaching approach, which includes a rare sensitivity to the human needs of people with Alzheimer's, along with an acute awareness of the frustrations of people trying to meet those needs.

As a specialist in rehabilitative medicine, I have worked with both adults and children with a range of neurologic disabilities. Planning home care for these individuals is often exceedingly difficult. Families need intensive guidance and support, and very few professionals have devoted the creative energy needed to provide families with a structured approach to coping with the stresses of caregiving.

The Alzheimer's Sourcebook opens a gateway for the future of caregiving. It describes an approach in which support and care become an organic, constantly adapting process, not a series of actions, but an art and a science of relationship, which grows from needs and issues of the family gathering around its afflicted member. This book shows how caregiving itself brings growth, a process in which everyone can gain and in which disease is not a villain, but a simple fact to be accommodated and, in the end, transcended as the family pursues a better quality of life for all.

The Alzheimer's Sourcebook offers hope by helping families see caregiving as a journey to be undertaken with intelligence, skill, and caring, not only for the benefit of our loved one, but for ourselves as well. Frena once told me that her main intention in this work was to provide light for a dark space. I believe that she has done exactly that.

Janet Lord, M.D.

Preface

I became involved with Alzheimer's disease in an entirely accidental way. I had just moved to the United States after twelve years of working in Asia as a journalist when the opportunity arose for me to become part of a caregiving team in Berkeley, California.

I lived in a house with four other amateur caregivers, whose task was to provide home-like care for a 79-year-old woman with Alzheimer's disease. Born in Germany, Hannah had been a promising young actress who was banned from the German stage by the Nazis. With her young husband, she fled to America—the only one of her immediate family to survive the concentration camps. Hannah raised her children, was widowed twice, earned her masters degree at the age of 64, and was diagnosed with Alzheimer's disease at the age of 75. This was the woman whose house I moved into.

I loved Hannah dearly. She was both loving and lovable, and she became the grandmother I had never known. I lived with her for a year, sharing her care with three others who knew as little about Alzheimer's disease as I did. Hannah was our teacher.

Up until then, I had been completely ignorant of Alzheimer's. When I left England in 1974, no one was talking about the disease. When I lived in Asia, it was not a topic I had ever heard about. I now recognize how blessed I was in knowing nothing.

If I had read all the comments that people routinely make about Alzheimer's disease today, perhaps I would have been too repelled, scared, or overwhelmed to think of becoming involved with it. My ignorance saved me from that bigotry.

Instead, I learned from Hannah. I learned that even if a person was greatly impaired, she could be fun and loving. Even if she needed a lot of attention, life could be interesting and varied. Even if she never learned my name—and Hannah was never able to remember my name—I always knew that I had a place in her heart. For a year, we made Hannah the center of our lives and our shared purpose was to help her lead as happy and stress-free of a life as possible. We tried every way we could to find out more about this disease, but everything we read or heard was dark, negative, and largely unhelpful. The only real help came from talking with other caregivers and learning from their experiences. And, I began to understand that the medical world had very little help to offer us.

Since there were four of us, Hannah had four different lives, plus the remains of her own, and she was a happy woman. The experience of becoming a caregiver completely transformed my own inner life, and I became deeply involved with the journey that caregivers undertake when they become Alzheimer's companions.

Knowing nothing, I learned from people who had Alzheimer's disease. I sat with them, talked with them, held them, sang to them, teased and amused them, wiped away their tears, and listened and watched. They have been my teachers, and they are still my teachers. They have taught me what they need, what they yearn for, and, how in the midst of all their losses, they can still grow. Because I learned from people who have Alzheimer's what the disease is all about, I do not devalue, dismiss, or diminish their experience. I know about the sense of separation, loneliness, and abandonment they feel. I also know they can still enjoy life, and there can be a whole of happiness even after Alzheimer's has begun.

This seems the right place to honor those teachers of mine: Hannah, my first and dearest teacher; Sheila Moon, the poet and psychoanalyst who was able to talk about the profound journey she was undertaking even in the depths of her Alzheimer's disease; and Janet Weinstein, a woman of great humor and character who faced her illness with the courage and determination to live life on her own terms.

I believe we are about to enter a new stage in our relationship with Alzheimer's disease. As a society we can no longer turn away from it. It is the great disease of the twentieth century, which challenges our fears and exposes the gaps in the cloth of our lives. We are going to have to stop talking about symptoms and begin relating to the people who have this disease. Only by doing so, will we find the answers that keep us from despair and bring light to our own journey. Only by taking the trouble to love will we find that there is something in this ordeal which can actually provide hope and spiritual help.

In this updated edition, I've included the latest information on research, medication, and the future of medical treatment, as well as information about the new gene test for diagnosing the disease.

It is not that Alzheimer's itself has any meaning. Illness just happens to someone, and that someone may be someone you know. The only part of the journey that can contain meaning is our journey to find the answer to the questions: What am I asked to learn? How am I to cope?

In traveling the road, we find answers to those questions, and out of that struggle comes some sense of meaning. This book is intended to be a guide to the journey, a light for the dark places, and a little hope for the times of despair.

CHAPTER 1

The Caregiver's Journey

....

If you've picked up this book, it's probably because someone you know has Alzheimer's disease or you suspect they do. You may be scared—angry too. You're terrified of the future. You've heard horrible things about Alzheimer's disease. You wonder how you're going to cope. And deep inside perhaps you wonder if it could happen to you. You want answers, even though you aren't sure what the questions should be.

This isn't the place to say "don't worry" or "relax." You probably can't do either right now. However, this is the place to say you are not alone. You are on a journey and this book will guide you through many of the more difficult passages. Others have been there before you and have found many different ways to cope. So will you. Knowledge will give you confidence, and experience will teach you how much you already know. You will have hard days, but you will also have many happy times. Life is not over because a person has Alzheimer's disease. There will still be adventures, rewards, laughter, and, of course, worry and anger and tears. Let us go together along this pathway you probably never wanted to take and share our time and the wisdom gathered from hundreds of caregivers all over America.

Being a caregiver is a profound spiritual and emotional journey for which most of us are unprepared. Most of us do not willingly become caregivers. It happens because a disaster overtakes someone we care about or feel responsible for. Looking after a person with Alzheimer's disease is a leap into the maelstrom of caregiving. You meet all kinds of turbulence, unexpected things happen, you develop skills you did not know you had. It is truly a journey into the unknown.

1

The caregiver's journey is unfamiliar to most of us. In all the new awarenesses brought to us by the psychological self-help movement, the caregiving of others has been the most neglected of all self-explorations. In fact, with the general recognition that unhealthy caring for others has been at the root of many negative family patterns, we have overlooked the importance of developing the skills of healthy caregiving.

Caregiving has become unfashionable, although it was normal in family life in the past. In previous ages, the sick usually stayed at home and certainly died there, ideally surrounded by family members, friends, and neighbors who accompanied them on the last great human journey up to the gates of death itself. It was the rare human being who never had the experience of caring for another in sickness, and even more rare for a person to have never been present at a death. These were once essential passages in adjusting to the demands of life, sickness, and death. By contrast, in this century there has been a massive movement toward placing the sick and dying in hospital care.

For a few decades, from the 1940s to the 1980s, the place for the dying was considered to be in a hospital, not at home. This is still the reality of the general pattern of care, but it is changing, largely in response to Western hospitals' incapacity to meet the real needs of the dying and their families, or even to acknowledge the reality and inevitability of death. Many people, once again, are opting to die where their life has been most meaningful—at home.

This slow return to a previous way of dealing with death and dying comes at a time when many people have become unfamiliar with caregiving. Fewer people have children. Most people go to hospitals when they are sick and stay in them to die, or go to nursing homes for their closing years or months of life. Many people have jobs that mean they cannot be available to care for another person at home. This means few have a chance to care for another person whose illness has made normal life impossible.

This book will help you to understand healthy caregiving. It will teach you how to cope and find solutions and how to find meaning and purpose in the caregiving journey, even in the profoundly difficult task of becoming a companion and caregiver to a person with Alzheimer's disease. Even with this dreaded disease, there are rewards to be found in caregiving and there is worth and fulfillment within the struggle.

Right now, of course, you just want to know more about Alzheimer's disease and get some ideas on coping with it. You want a few key facts that will magically enable you to become an effective caregiver and take away the problems of your daily life. However, you will soon find out—if you have not already—that just learning facts about this particular disease is not enough.

You already know that your doctor and your social worker and your neurologist cannot necessarily help you find the answers to daily life problems. Only the collective experience of many caregivers can do that. That is the knowledge and understanding that this book offers you on your journey. This book has been written by one caregiver with eight years of living and working with Alzheimer's disease who has also distilled the experiences of hundreds of other caregivers. It will show you what we all have learned from our encounters with Alzheimer's disease.

Even this is not the end of your exploration. It is true that finding approaches to solving problems is essential if you are to have any peace in your daily life. However, there is something more that will make your task meaningful and help you overcome the despair that weighs down so many Alzheimer caregivers. To meet this challenge successfully, you need to explore the profound meaning of this journey. Otherwise, you will succumb to the debilitating anger and depression that weighs down the people who regard this only as a cruel and meaningless affliction.

This is not to say that anyone recommends Alzheimer's disease as a rewarding undertaking. However, you cannot face the journey day after day if you get locked into despair or hopelessness that consumes your energy. You will miss the small pleasures and delights that can come when you spend time in that Alice-in-Wonderland world of someone with Alzheimer's disease. You will miss the areas in which an afflicted person can actually grow despite the illness. Noticing that growth and appreciating it helps reduce stress for you as the caregiver and for the person with Alzheimer's. It helps you focus on what is positive and allows you to show appreciation for who that person is now, instead of being locked into mourning who that person used to be.

You are undoubtedly familiar with many attitudes that surround Alzheimer's disease. Commonly, people describe it as horrible, degrading, and appalling. They often describe the person who has it as "dead," even when that person is sitting next to them. These attitudes cause much of the emotional attrition of this disease. It is the constant message that all is lost—that this disease is cruel and demeaning, that essentially it cannot be coped with—which overwhelms caregivers.

This book has been written to help you understand what the deeper elements of this disease mean to us as human beings, what growth is possible, and what personal development and spiritual strength come from bringing all your compassion, creativity, sense of humor, and ability to each day of living with Alzheimer's disease.

The Chinese say, when you cannot change a situation, then you have to change your mind. This book will help you to see that even the hardest situations give us some choices about how we deal with them. Right now, the Alzheimer situation cannot be changed, though we can hope the future will be different as medical science tackles the complexities of this disease and unravels its secrets. Right now, you must learn to live with it. To do that you may have to make some significant changes in your life.

Since so much of what you read and hear about Alzheimer's disease is negative, here are some positive items of information:

- Many people with Alzheimer's disease become much more open emotionally, showing affection and love as they never did before.
- The human journey to inward peace and resolution still continues for the person with Alzheimer's disease, and achieving happiness is entirely possible.
- As a caregiver, you can become a valuable part of that journey, both in helping the person you care for and in pursuing your own pathway.
- Many people with totally fragmented short-term memory function have astonishingly accurate long-term memory.

Therefore Alzheimer's disease does not preclude the final coming-to-terms with the primary relationships in life that is a normal part of the aging process for many older people.

Even people who are seriously impaired with dementia are often still clearly involved with this process of trying to find resolution. This is why they will ask to see their mothers and fathers (long dead) or why they sometimes wait for their parents to visit them. All human beings are somewhat in thrall to the shadow of their parents, alive or dead. The death of parents does not, by any means, release the child from patterns of need and reaction. Memory problems often cause people with Alzheimer's disease to forget that their parents are dead, but for them, as for the rest of us, parents are never truly dead. Therefore, the issue of finding peace can be very much a part of Alzheimer's disease.

Sometimes, persons with Alzheimer's repeat stories of old traumas and heartbreaks again and again, in an attempt to bring resolution to unhappy or frightening memories. Once you understand this as a caregiver, you can help the person you look after to reach a state of acceptance and letting go of the past. It will also help you to see that this is part of the meaning of this difficult passage in life.

This is one aspect of the journey that has been unexplored in the literature on the disease. In fact, persons with Alzheimer's disease and their caregivers have suffered a great deal from the silences regarding the small areas of hope and growth that surround them. We need to know about these positive aspects so that we can appreciate and encourage them.

- People with Alzheimer's also often keep certain special abilities they had—singers still sing, musicians still play, the spiritual will still be spiritually awake, although they will need more feeling and less intellectual ambiance for their spirituality.
- Pleasures are still pleasures—eating good food, enjoying flowers, delighting in small children, loving animals.
- The sense of humor remains.
- The awareness of sexuality—even the ability to flirt—often remains.

The purpose of reminding you about all this is that often we are so caught up in what people can no longer do that we forget to acknowledge and enjoy what they can do.

Some persons with Alzheimer's actually develop new ways to be creative, which is a true triumph of the human spirit. People who have never painted before can be led into painting with the right teacher. Group poetry-making can be a successful and moving venture. Music is a powerful communication tool that still speaks clearly to the impaired.

In the emotional range, many dementia-impaired people become more openly loving, more accepting of love, and more appreciative of tenderness and care. Emotional capacity becomes more naked in those who no longer have the mind structure to create barriers to hide their feelings. In many ways, the deepest revelation of the Alzheimer journey is that it is a kind of passage from the mind into the heart.

For the caregiver, one of the great teachings of this journey is that it reveals to us that a person is still fully a person even when impaired in memory and mental function. It demonstrates daily that love is always important.

Love, in fact, will be the greatest basis of all your skills. For some of you, this idea will be a relief because you already know you love the person you care for. If you feel despair or a sense of doom because you have troubled or unresolved feelings toward the person—for example, your mother was a lousy mother but now needs you to act as her good mother—don't give up. This book will help you unravel some of those tangles too. Resolution and forgiveness are possible for everyone willing to do the personal work needed. For other caregivers, such as spouses of people with Alzheimer's, personal growth and resolution come with accepting a change of role and forgiveness of the losses caused by this disease.

Once we learn to accept things as they are in the present moment—and we can learn to do that—everything else becomes possible.

These are the issues of the caregiver's journey. In our society today we often value people for what they do or have and usually much less for what they are. If we judge people to be damaged in any way, especially damaged in mind, we attach even less value to them. It is very hard for us to accept that every person is a valuable person and that every person has a deep and abiding need to be loved. Unfortunately, we tend to treat the impaired as less of a person and therefore as less lovable. We also treat him or her as less deserving of being treated as a whole person and as less needing of such treatment. Commonly, we hear people say that the person with Alzheimer's disease becomes like a child, and often the people around them treat them that way.

No one who is past the age of 11 is a child. An 80-year-old woman with severe dementia is an 80-year-old woman with all the experiences, dreams, hopes, and disappointments that go with long life. She may need us to communicate with her at the primary functioning level of a small child, but she also needs, and has a right to be respected as an adult. The good caregiver will do both. By using your understanding, you will learn to see the person as she or he really is.

People do not become simpler with Alzheimer's disease. They become more complex, and we need a complexity of skills to relate to them. Relationship is the center of the caregiver's journey. The average person with Alzheimer's usually does not need much nursing, or indeed may not need any. The unrelenting need is for companionship, understanding, compassion, supervision—oh yes, and love.

You probably understand by now why the path of the caregiver is a spiritual journey. This journey asks of us that we accept another person as always whole in spirit, as needing our unconditional love, and as being valued here and now as the person he or she is. When we only hark back to who this person used to be, we cause anguish for ourselves and create continuing anguish for the person with Alzheimer's disease. Many special moments are available in the here and now if we let go of the person we wish someone to be.

In the case of a caregiver who is a family member, this means letting go of mother as a mother or husband as a spouse. This is hard and painful to do, but if we cannot do it, we create more pain every minute of our day. We must also forgive the person, and the list of items up for forgiveness may well be extensive. We must:

- Forgive the illness and its symptoms.
- Forgive any wrongs that person did us in the past.
- Forgive for never being able to have things "right" again.
- Forgive for the plans we made that have been spoiled.
- Forgive the forgetting.
- Forgive that person whose illness constantly reminds us how we fail as caregivers.
- Forgive ourselves for the ways we fail as caregivers.

What is good about this journey for the caregiver? It teaches us many of the deepest spiritual truths in everyday life. No sitting alone in a forest clearing for the Alzheimer caregiver. No, it is unremitting daily life experience that brings the caregiver to the exact same place that the forest meditator eventually hopes to come to—the place of unconditional love.

There is nothing ethereal, otherworldly, or wishy-washy about this love. Unconditional love does not mean perfect behavior, nor is it sentimental. It is basic, real, connected, and ordinary—that is what makes it extraordinary, of course. You will receive constant cueing about how you are relating to the person you look after. In Alzheimer's, although there can be confusion and bewilderment on both the part of the caregiver and the person with the illness, nevertheless certain things will always be very clear. The person you look after will become your teacher in those things.

When you are angry, even if you hide it from yourself, your anger will be reflected back by the person with Alzheimer's. When you are anxious, hurried, or brusque, that person responds with loss of function, bizarre behavior, or confusion, and uncertainty. You are accountable for everything you feel because it brings response. You will get to know yourself probably better than you wanted to. The enormous plus in all this is that you can be exactly who you are with the person who has Alzheimer's. You will always be accepted as you are because memory loss removes expectation and the ability to recollect your failings. You can be silly or emotional or irritable and you will always be forgiven because it will always be forgotten. This is a giant spiritual gift because, through another person's forgetting, you will forgive yourself. You get to start afresh all the time with a person who has Alzheimer's disease. Each day is a new beginning. You can regard that as a curse or as a blessing. If you are wise, you will work with it as a blessing.

You will discover the power of love each moment because it is the best practical way to make life work with Alzheimer's. A mistake? You give a hug. Fear? You give a hug. Anxiety? You give a backrub. Restlessness? Make a joke and give a hug. Love will become your most reliable management technique.

If this begins to sound as if you have to do all the giving, certainly there is an element of truth to that. However, if you continue to learn to be a good caregiver, you will also learn to receive. Get a hug, get a backrub, share some of your sadness. The person with Alzheimer's is perfectly capable of giving and sharing. You do not have to always stand alone. Although it is true that the disease causes great losses that probably make you feel sad and sometimes very lonely, still there are many times you could share being together. These might not be in the ways you want, but that is where you just have to accept what is. Usually you can find ways to be less alone.

You can be completely honest. You can say that you feel angry or frustrated or lonely and it will not be held against you. Honesty works well in Alzheimer's. In fact, it is the best possible policy. Later chapters will show you how to communicate well and how to understand what is being communicated to you, but meanwhile know that honesty works as one of your best tools.

Perhaps the deepest spiritual lesson in all of this is that unless we tend our own needs we cannot tend to another's. Caregivers who do not look after themselves often become inadequate caregivers because they have exhausted their inner resources. We must ask so that we can receive. One person alone cannot deal with Alzheimer's. It is false pride to think so. It is not even fair to try since it will mean poor caregiving and even lead to abuse of the person who is sick.

We have to ask others for help, and in that way we open pathways for others to show love. Often, outsiders can be more loving, and accepting than family caregivers can, because the outsider does not have the psychic history that the family carries. The caregiver who rejects help from others, who insists on standing alone, who wants to control the whole situation, only comes to exhaustion and despair. This is the typical overachieving caregiver who fills Alzheimer literature, and is the most commonly seen figure in Alzheimer stories in the media.

Up to now, society has stood back to watch this overachiever with respect and awe, assuming this must be the true picture of Alzheimer care. However, this image does not serve anyone well. It is time to stop applauding overachieving in caregiving because it leads to bad caregiving and destroys both giver and receiver. Many of the so-called problem behaviors of Alzheimer's come from situations where overachieving caregivers are trying to maintain control. This is not to criticize but just to gently indicate that it is time to let go of that damaging stereotype and work toward real health in caregiving, just as we are seeking health in other dependent relationships in our society. There is nothing noble about a person who becomes ill with caregiving. It is a tragic waste of human effort and caring. This book will teach you how to avoid the traps of becoming an overachieving caregiver and help you to plan your outreach for help.

Caregiving teaches us, finally, that human beings need love all the way to the gates of death and that love always matters. Often families fade out of the scene once someone is in full-time care. They say, "She doesn't even know me," when the issue is not knowing but loving. Someone who cannot intellectually get your name right still needs love. Moreover, if we really try to understand Alzheimer's, then we come to realize that when your mother calls you "Mother," it is not that she has forgotten your role as her daughter, it is that she needs your maternal love in her sickness, and does, in fact, recognize you as deeply important.

If we can take the risk of feeling our pain, and our loss, then we can be free to love as much as is needed—that is, unconditionally. If we can face the terror of the disease that is most feared by most people in the United States today, then we can be free to love instead of running away. When we can go to the nursing home to see Grandma, and hold her hand even if she cannot acknowledge our ego needs, then we are demonstrating exactly what family is supposed to be about. After all, if the family does not supply Grandma's need for love, who exactly is supposed to be there fulfilling that need?

When we give our full accepting love in the here and now moment, we learn that the average person with Alzheimer's can experience a lot of happiness in an average day. It is true that Alzheimer's strikes at the roots of our terror of depending upon others, and not getting enough love. However, it is not on the whole a physically painful disease. The most emotionally difficult stages for people with the disease are usually the early stages. Later on, with the right caregivers around, daily life can be very pleasant. Many people in the later stages enter a kind of blissfulness in which it is obvious that they have reached resolution. While there may be times when the person becomes agitated, this usually does not last long. It passes, and is not remembered. People with Alzheimer's do not hold on to what distresses or frightens them in the moment. The blessing of the disease is the same as the curse—forgetfulness.

The real anguish of this disease is carried by family members and also by those who have never been around it. This anguish is caused by the psychic input from the world that says this is surely the most terrible disease there is. That attitude comes mainly from those who do not understand the disease and from those caregivers who do not take care of themselves and therefore become depressed, dysfunctional, and despairing. Much of this despair is a by-product of lack of sleep and failure to deal honestly with feelings.

We need not dread Alzheimer's so much if we know that it causes little physical pain and that its emotional pain can often be greatly alleviated by good caregiving. If we do not feel the disease is demeaning, the sufferer is freed from feeling demeaned. So it helps if we let go of some of our own judgments about this illness.

The bright side for you as the caregiver is that, even if you never wanted to be a caregiver—and still do not want to but are obliged to for family or personal reasons—you can learn to do it well, and you will reap all the spiritual and emotional benefits. You may also incur all the immense emotional costs too, so be sure to read all the chapters in this book that will help you with details, and problems. If you dislike the word spiritual, ignore it, and just do the job well anyway. You will still get many benefits. If you think it is insulting to have to read about love when you want to read only the latest information on Alzheimer treatment, that's okay.

Read these chapters, get on with caregiving, and check in again in a few weeks' time to see if love is any part of your agenda yet. It may not matter to anyone else if you do not deal with the issues of love in your life, but it will matter to the person with Alzheimer's disease, and that person will let you know about it in a thousand subtle and not so subtle ways.

If you are a caregiver or about to become one, congratulations! You are joining a little band of warriors who are not deeply appreciated in this world where examinations, technology, and documentation have taken over the world of caregiving but have left many people who need loving care bereft and alone. The home caregiver is one of the great unsung heroes of today. If you are one, know that there are many others like you. You will find them at support group meetings all over the country—brave people living the ordinary life in extraordinary ways.

You have chosen, or have had thrust upon you, one of the great human journeys. As an Alzheimer companion, you have elected to accompany another human being into one of the most mysterious pathways of the human spirit. You will be the light for someone else's darkness. You will have to walk through what is still a scarcely-known underworld, the shadowside of memory. This book will help you enormously on that journey with all the facts and practical information, and how-to techniques, but you already have the only real weapon needed against the shadows.

The name of the weapon is Love.

CHAPTER 2

Before Diagnosis

....

"Looking back, I can see now that Dad's illness started years before. He stopped going out to play cards with his buddies. He always used to go every Friday night, but gradually he began not bothering. I asked him why and he said he just didn't want to, but I suppose it was because he couldn't manage the game any more and didn't want to say so. It was his secret. Over the next few years, he let more and more of his old life go. He even stopped driving. He said he couldn't see any more, but I think that was just his excuse," says Ken, whose father is 75 and has Alzheimer's disease.

Many times, long before a person is actually diagnosed as having Alzheimer's disease, there are small indicators of something wrong. These signs often puzzle or alarm family members, but until they have accumulated sufficiently to cause major disquiet, their real significance is not really understood. Only in looking back are they seen as signposts of Alzheimer's.

As one family member put it, "Mom was always a bit strange, to be honest. She had her odd ways which we kids all just thought of as being Mom's personal style. For example, one thing she did was to dry paper towels over a toaster. She did it for years and we didn't really even know it was strange at the time. We just knew this was what Mom did. Of course, now that she's been diagnosed with Alzheimer's, we often ask ourselves if this was a very early sign and no one knew it."

Since dementia takes many forms, it is hard to list all the questionable behaviors that may indicate its presence. Even if we could list them all, we could not be sure what they signified.

"We thought Grandma was just upset after Grandpa died. She wouldn't go out. She didn't have her hair done any more. We always used to have big Sunday lunches at Grandma's house and she did all the cooking, but then she said she couldn't be bothered any more. Then bailiffs came from the sheriff's office and Dad found she hadn't paid any property taxes for years. He found all the bills in a drawer. She nearly lost the house," says Adam, whose grandmother was diagnosed at 69 with Alzheimer's disease.

A whole range of odd behaviors make up each person's idiosyncratic style. If we later develop Alzheimer's, our own families will not know whether to attribute these idiosyncrasies to our disease or to our personal styles of being. Most Alzheimer indicators are behaviors that accumulate until they actually interfere with normal life; until they do interfere with a person's functioning, we cannot claim them as indicators of Alzheimer's disease. In fact, it is important that we do not. It will become clear as you read on that the so-called Alzheimer symptoms can be signs of many other conditions; some may be caused by medications (the average older person is taking six medications at any one time). Therefore, be alert to possible warning signs but do not make any assumptions.

Experts in the Alzheimer field warn us that many older people with various problems are categorized as having Alzheimer's disease when in fact they do not. This particular dementia has become a catch-all basket into which all kinds of cases are thrown, including conditions that could well be treated. Residing in every Alzheimer's care unit are people suspected by the staff of not having Alzheimer's at all and who have never been formally diagnosed. Even the medical profession makes this mistake, so it is obvious that self-appointed amateur Alzheimer-spotters only confuse things further.

No amateur can accurately classify a symptom. Even medical experts can do so only with extensive testing. In fact, the final diagnosis of Alzheimer's disease is made only after all other possibilities have been eliminated. It is a diagnosis that basically says, "We can't find anything else that fits, so we can reasonably assume that what we are left with must be Alzheimer's disease." The diagnosis is usually stated to be "a dementia of the

Alzheimer's type," sometimes shortened to DAT. If someone you know exhibits a number of the signs and symptoms discussed below, proper medical investigation is needed. These signs are warnings that something is wrong, whether that something is depression or liver disease or Alzheimer's disease.

Also be aware that every individual with Alzheimer's has a personal style of presenting the disease. These variations cause confusion and questions among family members. Alzheimer's sufferers have certain universal problems, the most obvious being memory loss, but other symptoms vary widely, so much so that some medical experts are currently suggesting that there are several different kinds of Alzheimer's disease. Some think that this is not so much a specific disease as a collection of identifying behaviors and variable symptoms—in other words, a syndrome.

If you are worried about a family member who presents a number of these symptoms, encourage the person to get a complete checkup, including neurological testing, CAT scans, and laboratory tests. Beforehand, speak privately to the doctor about your concerns so that the doctor will include a dementia test while interviewing the patient and will be alert to possible cover-up of problems by the patient. It is typical for Alzheimer patients to deny there is anything wrong with them, often in a confident and convincing manner. Many family members report their frustration over this.

"I told the doctor my husband was having severe memory problems, but the doctor just asked him if he ever forgot anything and my husband said cheerfully, 'Oh no, in fact I've got a great memory.' Frankly, I could have killed the pair of them!" reports one frustrated wife.

It was a year later before her husband was finally diagnosed, and that was only after she had insisted on a full Alzheimer workup from a neurologist. Some families have communication problems with their doctors over their early suspicions. Some physicians shrug off the concerns by vague phrases like, "What can you expect at his age?" or "There may be a little senility there." There are many good doctors and it is essential to have one when dealing with Alzheimer's, even if this means changing your doctor. Since Alzheimer's is so variable, you need an experienced doctor to deal with it.

15

Those who work with many Alzheimer sufferers and talk with their families recognize that there is a much earlier phase than the one normally identified as "early stage." This is the "invisible phase." It covers the period of time—that could extend for many years—in which only the individual concerned knows or suspects there is something wrong. One woman, diagnosed at 74, had written in her diaries 20 years before that she was experiencing problems with her thinking. She had what she called "these terrible absentmindednesses of mine," that involved both memory lapses and problems in thinking things through. Another woman, a highly regarded Jungian psychologist, noted a series of dreams she had 30 years before being diagnosed with Alzheimer's disease in which doctors told her she had an incurable brain disease. She did not interpret these dreams literally at the time and it was only her later illness that retrospectively suggested that she should have.

Many anecdotes like this suggest interesting questions about how some people have a deep inner knowledge of their true state of health, even before any are visible signs of illness are present.

The Invisible Phase, during which the individual lives privately with the growing awareness that something is wrong, is seen by others only in behavior changes, often inexplicable at the time. An outgoing, gregarious man gave up his social life entirely, telling his wife he just could not be bothered. At the time, she put it down to the demands of his work, but later she saw it as the beginning of Alzheimer's disease. Another woman stopped playing mahjongg with her friends. When her son asked her why, she answered vaguely, "Oh, I don't like those people any more." Other people show no outward signs that they are troubled and yet later discoveries reveal that they were aware of their encroaching illness. One woman started collecting articles on memory loss dating from her early forties, even though she worked at a demanding job until normal retirement age and was not actually diagnosed until she was 80. Her family discovered her secret cache of cuttings after she went into skilled nursing care.

Other signs are much more outward. A man who never drank to excess began to drink heavily and to throw temper tantrums at home. This period extended for several years, during which his wife was frantic. "I thought Bill hated me. I thought he was going to leave me. He used to scream at me and throw his dinner plate against the walls. I had no idea what was going on at that time." When Bill was finally identified as having Alzheimer's disease, his wife understood that he had been reacting in sheer terror to his knowledge that he was losing control within.

Either because of denial or simply because he did not know the nature of what was going on, Bill never spoke about his fears to his wife. When he was finally diagnosed and the doctor broke the news to him and his wife together, Bill said, "Thank God! Oh, thank God! I thought I was going crazy!" This is not an uncommon reaction among Alzheimer sufferers. While their families are afraid to mention the word Alzheimer's to them, they themselves are often convinced that they are going mad or becoming stupid. They cannot talk about their unformulated fears and feelings. Instead, they act them out.

Many behavior changes may mark the invisible phase:

- intense suspicion and fear of others
- outbursts of rage
- inability to follow through with projects
- problems following thoughts through
- the onset of depression
- the sudden start of drinking bouts in a person not previously given to drinking
- inability to continue responsibility in work, community, or family affairs
- curious inability to get hold of an idea or a thought process
- gaps of logic that cannot be filled no matter how often others explain them
- outbreaks of irrational rage
- responding with hostility for no apparent reason
- unbelievable stories of bad things done by others

All of these signs could indicate problems with thought processes and the gradual failure of rational thinking ability, together with emotional attrition.

Often family members notice changes but cannot identify what they signify, either because they really do not know or because they are in denial. It is hard for families to admit that something is wrong. For a long time, individual members just harbor their secret suspicions.

"I noticed my mother started avoiding people, even family members," says Mary, whose 85-year-old mother lives in an Alzheimer care unit. "Once, her sister came to visit and my mother refused even to come out of her room the whole time her sister was there. Yet they'd always been close. It was really embarrassing and I didn't understand it at all. Maybe she didn't want anyone to know there was something wrong with her and she thought her sister would notice."

Often, the only sign of trouble is a mood change—depression, anxiety, or increasing dependence even over very small things. These lead to greater emotional stress for both family members and for the person who is finally manifesting the first visible signs of disease. One woman of 74 was told by her youngest son to become more independent at a time when, unknown to him, she was reminding herself who her own children were by writing memos in her diary: "My youngest son is Myron and he teaches high school students. My oldest son is Deiter and he's a doctor in Chicago." Her sudden extra dependency came out of her knowledge that she was losing her memory.

Another family identified their mother's early dementia as "Mother's nerves" and explained her tears and tantrums as a sign that she and their father were not enjoying their retirement. As true as that observation was, it was far from being the real story. They tried to deal with their mother's growing incapacity by bringing in household help, except that their mother would fire the help behind their backs. She was not ready to reveal her neediness other than to family members, who in turn were not ready to acknowledge it.

Thus, although the common medical term for the cumulative gathering of visible symptoms is early stage Alzheimer's, we can now see that this is not necessarily a correct description of how far the disease has progressed. Family members must not think this term literally means the disease is in its beginnings.

After the invisible stage comes the "visible early stage." During this time, which again may extend for many years or a few months, the family sees a number of disquieting signs. They are likely to include some or all of the following:

- overall inability to function as well as before
- deterioration in appearance
- changes in grooming and dress
- wearing slightly odd combinations of clothing
- decline in personal hygiene
- incapacity to deal with household bills and documents
- dropping old friendships and social patterns
- becoming more dependent
- avoiding contact even with close family members
- staying in bed for long periods for no apparent reason
- becoming fearful or anxious for no apparent reason
- telling stories about neighbors doing bad things
- relating strange events
- calling the police for no valid reason
- having domestic accidents
- leaving pots burning on the stove
- leaving appliances on
- change in sleep patterns
- getting lost in the car or having a series of unaccounted-for car accidents
- being unable to account for the day's activities
- showing inconsistencies of memory or behavior
- lack of food in the refrigerator or cupboards
- hoarding one kind of food, such as 18 cans of beans or 8 packets of cookies
- mood changes seemingly unrelated to external events

This list could be endless, since any kind of variation might appear in any individual. Basically, these signs all add up to decreasing competency in daily life, increasing memory problems, and signs of emotional distress. Obviously, there are many possible reasons for these developments, which is why it is important to persuade the person to seek help.

This can be the hardest thing of all since most families tend to respect the desire of members to remain independent as long as possible. They do not want to interfere. However, in general, families intervene too late rather than too soon. It is almost unknown for a family to intervene inappropriately early. Be confident that by the time you have noticed signs of distress accumulating, you are dealing with an important problem.

Even when the whole family recognizes there is a problem, they often hesitate to interfere until the disease becomes much more advanced. If this is your case, it would be a good idea for all your family members to talk about how you can ensure life quality, tactful help, and discreet monitoring of the impaired person's lifestyle. Consider a shopping plan, a visiting plan, a meal schedule, help with household papers, and bills, and so on.

It is not a kindness to leave people with dementia to cope beyond their capacity to do so. It places a heavy burden on them and undoubtedly adds to their stress tremendously. Demented people cannot run their own lives. It is that simple. Of course, it is hard to know exactly how to intervene. Most people resent your butting in. Whatever their degree of stress, your own family members hardly ever say, "Why, yes thank you for suggesting I can't run my own life. I'm so grateful you want to take it over for me!"

Family members need to get together to discuss what they are seeing. Ideally, everyone makes an input into this discussion and it becomes a reality check for the whole family. This is important since the early visible stages of Alzheimer's are often somewhat nebulous—a fading of capacity rather than a clearly delineated set of circumstances.

It is helpful for everyone to make a list of the problems. Note down each incident or symptom and discuss whether this adds up to illness. Normal idiosyncrasies should be left off the list. For example, if Mother has always had unkempt hair, then this should not be listed. You are looking for changes that indicate a decline is going on, a growing inability to manage life as before. When only one or two indicators are found, assume that this slight decline is within the range of normal aging and stop worrying. If the list is long, obviously there are problems.

It is normal for people approaching their final years to show a certain amount of withdrawal from the things of everyday life. In our new awareness of Alzheimer's, we must not label all such withdrawals as dementia. A woman of 90 who begins to forget names and addresses from the present when she is inwardly concentrating upon setting her primary relationships to peace before death does not deserve the label of Alzheimer's disease.

Even if you have compiled a symptom list applying to your family member, this is not necessarily a reason to rush the ailing person into medical or nursing care. Increasing family support could help to keep the person coping with limited independence. Family members could take over certain household tasks and see whether the situation gets better, worse, or is holding at a plateau. Unless an actual trauma of some kind occurs, family members need not hurry into life-changing decisions.

When trauma occurs, however, rapid decline results. Almost every family story of Alzheimer's disease mentions that the major signs of decline come on quickly after trauma. People manage more or less for a long time, even with an accumulation of problems, then comes a sudden catastrophe. After that, seemingly, they become overwhelmed. Some researchers suggest that this may come about through a collapse of the immune system through the result of trauma.

Autopsy research has shown that the actual physical deterioration of the brain bears no relationship to the outward signs of dementia. A number of people, autopsied for other causes of death, have been found to have all the signs of severe Alzheimer's-like brain deterioration and yet showed no dementia behaviors. This suggests that the physical attack on the brain is not always the main factor in deterioration. The other factor lies in the mystery of human resistance to disease. When that collapses through stress, it is as if the disease suddenly runs on apace. This probably accounts for the family stories that say, "Mother was fine until Dad died. Then she suddenly got Alzheimer's disease."

The kinds of trauma that may lead to increased manifestations of possible Alzheimer's disease include the following:

• the death of a spouse, close family member, or good friend
• a change of residence
• a car accident, even with no injuries
• a fall, whether with injury or not
• surgery, especially under general anesthesia
• being the victim of threatened or actual violence, such as being mugged
• being the victim of a burglary
• retirement or the unwelcome loss of a job
• developing another serious illness
• emotional stress
• general failure to thrive, a term used normally only of infants and small children but equally applicable to older people undergoing adverse age changes or emotional reactions

There are a few physical indicators of possible Alzheimer's disease. These include the sudden development of intense sugar cravings, even in people who never liked sweet things before, and the loss of the sense of smell. We do not yet understand these factors although we can make guesses. Dietary researchers assert that the average person with Alzheimer's disease uses up some 4,000 calories per day, enough for heavy physical labor. This burning of calories, which may be due to the whole physical system being in overdrive merely to cope, probably accounts for the sugar cravings that are universal in dementia sufferers.

Other early signs are not in the person but in the environment, small clues that something is wrong.

"I kept finding sheets in the oven and when I asked Mom why they were there, she'd say she was drying them. That was the only thing, and after a while it even seemed fairly normal to me. I just thought, 'Oh yes, there's Mom's sheets in the oven again.' She didn't have it switched on, so there wasn't any danger," Mary recalls.

Finding things in strange places—matches in the freezer, clothes in the oven—indicates a shift in thought processes. Hearing stories that just do not add up or make sense; finding your family member cannot account for a day's activities at all; unaccustomed discrepancies in management of household finances, such as paying a bill several times, or not at all—all these indicate severe problems. Then there is the refrigerator test—the refrigerator of the average Alzheimer's patient contains one dried lemon, two eggs, several ancient containers of food from restaurants, and two gallons of chocolate ice cream.

These are only signs of distress if they represent a change in behavior and life management. If a woman has always hoarded food items, then 20 cans of corn in her cupboard do not necessarily represent Alzheimer's. The typical Alzheimer refrigerator could also be the typical young student's refrigerator, so the key again is whether a change in the environment has appeared.

Likewise, gradual decline in cleanliness of a house, management of a garden, or cooking ability are signs suggesting that something is wrong.

If you are a family member worried about someone and you find that much of this chapter applies, what do you do? If your relative admits the problem, that is one thing. If your relative refuses even to admit there is anything wrong, you have a serious dilemma. You may have to stand by for years before crisis offers a chance for intervention. Rather than worry about your frustration or fears, concentrate on what you can do. You can help where it is acceptable—spring cleaning, taking the person out for a meal, shopping. You can also join a support group. Many people who attend Alzheimer support groups are there because they suspect someone has dementia, not because they know.

Go to see your relative's doctor to express your worries. This will enable the doctor to be aware of possible memory and dementia issues when next examining your relative.

That, for the time being, is all you can do. Often, being a good friend to someone with Alzheimer's simply consists of acceptance, support, and love, with practical aid whenever it can be given and accepted. Try not to project your fears about

Alzheimer's on the person you suspect may have it. Instead, just be open to finding ways to be in that person's life that help both of you relate to each other. Someone who fears he or she has something wrong is much more likely to confide those fears in a trusted and loved friend or relative. So be prepared, if you know someone who shows a number of the signs mentioned in this chapter, to serve by standing and waiting.

Alzheimer's Disease: The Facts

....

Wisdom is the principal thing; therefore get wisdom: and with all thy getting, get understanding.

—PROVERBS 4:7

This chapter contains a picture of the full course of Alzheimer's disease: what we currently know about it, recent research, current uses of medication, and likely medical developments in its future treatment.

It is important to remember, however, that *everyone does Alzheimer's disease in a totally individual way.* Certain symptoms may be universal—memory problems, for example—but otherwise, there is great variation from person to person and even in one person from day to day. Therefore, do not assume that the typical course of the disease outlined here is what will happen to your parent. In fact, very few people live to the so-called last stages of Alzheimer's disease, although that is the picture most people imagine and dread on behalf of their own family member.

Alzheimer's disease is not a new disease, nor one confined to this century. In fact, the earliest documented mention of a condition that now looks like Alzheimer's disease was in 500 B.C. when Solon, the famous Greek lawyer and philosopher, wrote that impaired judgment from old age could cause a will to be invalid.

It is only our awareness which is new. One of the possible reasons why we hear so much about Alzheimer's disease is because of the huge increase in the number of people living longer. While the actual span of human life has not really extended, the percentage of people living to its extent has megajumped.

So, what we are now seeing is the disease process. Although current concentration on Alzheimer's disease may be frightening for some people, it actually has positive aspects. We now know, for example, that people in old age can reasonably expect good health. After all, if 10 percent of people age 65 have Alzheimer's, that means 90 out of every 100 do not. That is a pretty good set of figures.

Alzheimer's disease is perhaps the best-known, most-feared disease of this century. It is an organic brain disease of unknown cause. Alzheimer's is not classified as a mental illness, but a physical deterioration of the brain which disrupts normal mental processes. It sets up physical roadblocks throughout the entire brain, short-circuiting the message system which controls everyday functions and mental organization. Essentially, Alzheimer's causes the computer of the brain to go down, and the whole of life becomes gradually disarrayed.

The American Psychiatric Association's definition of Alzheimer's disease contained in the diagnostic manual *DSM-IV*, is as follows:

> *The essential feature of the presence of Dementia of insidious onset and gradual progressive course for which all other specific causes have been excluded by the history, physical examination, and laboratory tests.*
>
> *The Dementia involves a multifaceted loss of intellectual abilities, such as memory, judgment, abstract thought, and other higher cortical functions, and changes in personality and behavior.*

This deterioration disrupts the normal working of the brain and gives rise to the manifestations of Alzheimer's disease—the slow, progressive, and so far irreversible loss of brain functions.

The course of the disease has three stages: early (or first) stage, middle (or second) stage, and final (or third, last or terminal) stage.

There may also be an initial "invisible" stage, which is apparent only to the sufferer who is inwardly aware of frightening changes in memory process. However, it is hard to prove since this is also a stage of great denial.

In the early stage of the disease, a person typically has signs

26

of memory loss—forgetting names, events, day, and year—and may show some decline in intellectual ability, unable to learn new skills or procedures or carry out abstract tasks. If the person is still working, problems at work may appear, with a drop in performance or sudden early retirement. Some signs of personality change may begin—increased withdrawal, less enjoyment of daily pleasures, dropping previous routines—but these are likely to be subtle.

These difficulties increase as the person proceeds from early to middle stage, usually two to ten years after diagnosis. Typical of the second stage is the appearance of much more apparent memory problems—forgetting names of neighbors, family members and daily events.

There may be inability to understand what is going on, less ability to express things, lack of grooming, failure to keep up household routines, not paying bills, and an inability to manage money. It will be harder for the person in second stage to follow explanations and arguments, and this may look like stubbornness, but it is not.

Activities may be dropped altogether, without explanation—no longer reading, problems with writing, changes in physical posture and movement, and refusing to go out. Apparently irrational fears may develop: "The neighbors are stealing from me." Accidents keep happening—car accidents unaccounted for or blamed on others, pots left burning, appliances left on. Personality changes may occur: outbursts of anger, hostility, weeping, anxiety attacks, depression.

Much more noticeable signs will appear, and family members will probably become aware at this point, if not before, of a serious problem. In fact, this is when family intervention begins. However, there are no clearly-delineated differences between the early and middle stages because the individual pathway varies so much. Often, you may want to know for sure at what stage your parent is but receive an inaccurate answer from medical professionals. That's because there is no objective answer. Most of the time, people who are not in full-time care are somewhere along the spectrum of the second stage.

The last stage includes severe impairment, even the loss of the ability to speak, walk, and eat, and incontinence is possible.

Few, if any, people will be recognized. Again, although this is the official line, few people actually fulfill all those predictions.

The Alzheimer's Association says that over 4 million Americans currently have Alzheimer's disease, and the course of the disease runs anywhere from three to 26 years. Nine years is the median length of time. These figures, however, come from the date of diagnosis which may or may not bear any relationship to the emergence of the first stage of the illness. Although the disease is not actually considered to be one of old age—the youngest person ever diagnosed with Alzheimer's disease was only 27-years-old—most people who have Alzheimer's are over 65.

Ten percent of people age 65 may have Alzheimer's disease, the number rising with age. One study claims that up to 47 percent of persons age 85 and over will have Alzheimer's disease, but that seems a very questionable conclusion. If almost half the aged population has a disease, then Alzheimer's is not a disease but a normal condition of old age. So, perhaps we should wait for more and possibly better studies to confirm or deny this conclusion.

Who gets Alzheimer's disease? Just about anyone. It is found in all societies and in all classes and types of people all across the world, from the Western world to the South Sea Islands, to China, India, and Japan. There are some variations in its groupings; a lower incidence in Japan; a very high incidence in the Marshall Islands; and more women than men, but this may only be a reflection of the fact that women live to a greater age than men. Early-onset Alzheimer's disease may be seen as early as a person's forties and fifties. The younger a person is at diagnosis, the greater the tendency is for the disease to run shorter and harder.

Alzheimer's disease is named after the German doctor Alois Alzheimer, who made a study of dementia after starting out as a clinician interested in nervous and mental diseases. He wanted to find the physical origins of dementia.

As both a practicing physician and a researcher, Dr. Alzheimer became known for his expertise in bringing together what information he had from his patients' lives and the results of brain autopsy to make important new discoveries in the study of dementia.

Using a newly developed, high-resolution microscope, Dr. Alzheimer found evidence of brain deterioration in those patients diagnosed with dementia. He found a pattern of damage which is still considered to be the clue to the presence of Alzheimer's disease during autopsy: large numbers of senile plaques and fibrillary tangles in the brain cells. These were the visible signs of degeneration in the nerve endings and the reason why the person became so impaired in functioning. Alzheimer thought that this microscopic evidence proved the presence of disease, but it was his superior and sponsor Dr. Emil Kraepelin who named this Alzheimer's disease in his own clinical textbook published in 1910.

Dr. Alzheimer's own conclusions about his discovery are not shared by doctors today. He thought he had found the cause of pre-senile dementia, a dementia which appeared before the age of 65. He considered that dementias which appeared after age 65 were due to vascular factors and should be called "senile dementia." Today, doctors do not make those particular divisions. They consider both early-onset dementias and dementias developing after age 65 to be Alzheimer's disease. The term senile dementia merely means "old-age dementia," and it can include dementias with a variety of causes, some temporary and curable, others irreversible. It is a term used loosely by doctors.

Dr. Alzheimer made his discovery in the late 1890s and, in 1907, wrote up his keynote case of a 51-year-old woman brought to see him by her husband. She suffered various impairments and died within the year. Dr. Alzheimer conducted an autopsy of her brain and discovered the benchmark plaques and tangles. However, it was not until the late 1960s that the term Alzheimer's disease was used.

About 50 percent of cases of late-life dementia are considered to be due to Alzheimer's disease. About 15 percent of cases are due to vascular factors and called Multi-Infarct Dementia (due to many small strokes). Another 25 percent of dementias are considered to be due to mixed degenerative and vascular factors (both Alzheimer's and Multi-Infarct), and are termed "mixed dementias." Dementia also can result from Parkinson's disease, or as a part of late Parkinson's disease; in Pick's disease and Creutzfeldt-Jacob disease (both rare); and memory loss, but not general dementia, comes from Korsakoff's syndrome (resulting from long-term alcohol abuse). The final 10 percent of dementias are considered to be of entirely unknown origin.

The term "organic brain syndrome," sometimes used by doctors as a diagnosis, is a general term which comes from the *DSM*—the bible of definitions issued by the American Psychiatric Association. Organic brain syndrome has little specific meaning, other than to say that dementia is present due to causes unspecified by this extremely generalized and, therefore, not very useful term.

If your parent has been diagnosed as having Alzheimer's disease, you probably have two great wishes. One, for the cure, and two, to know the cause. There is currently no cure, although a great deal of research is being done, which we discuss later. The news is not much better when it comes to considering the cause or causes. Right now, we have no idea what causes most cases of Alzheimer's disease. Researchers are exploring the following important avenues of inquiry:

BRAIN RESEARCH

a) *Neurotransmitters* are the chemical messengers of the brain, some of which fail their duties in Alzheimer's disease. The particular failures found so far are deficiencies in acetylcholine, with additional problems identified in somatostatin, norepinephrine, serotonin, and corticotrophin-releasing factors.

Researchers are experimenting in supplying the missing chemical to see if function can be restored and, if so, how permanently. Studies are promising. For example, lack of serotonin is connected with sleeplessness. Therefore, giving serotonin to people with Alzheimer's may be the answer to nighttime restlessness.

b) *Abnormal proteins:* Amyloid proteins are found in abnormal quantities in the brains of people with Alzheimer's, and the production of this protein is associated with chromosome 21. Researchers are trying to discover why amyloid is produced in these greater quantities and whether the process can be reduced.

ALUMINUM

Aluminum has been found in abnormal quantities in the brains of people with Alzheimer's, though various studies have not yet clarified whether this is a cause or merely a disease by-product.

Newer research also shows larger-than-normal deposits of iron in the brains of people with Alzheimer's, which indicates a connection between the quantity of zinc in the brain and Alzheimer's. Again, we do not yet know whether these are causes or side effects of the dementia.

Many people ask if they should stop using aluminum products. No one knows the answer, so it may not hurt. However, you are exposed to aluminum more than you might think—deodorants, drinking water, antacids, soft drink packaging. You might also reduce your intake of iron supplements and replace them with foods that are iron-rich instead.

GENETICS

There are two aspects to this question, heredity and genetics. A disorder can be hereditary, which means it runs in the family, but not necessarily genetic, which is due to prenatal factors. Both aspects are being explored in Alzheimer's research.

If your parent has Alzheimer's disease, you will of course worry whether you will develop it. However, there is very little evidence to suggest that the disease is hereditary. Only in very rare instances is there a definite genetic link, and that applies to only a handful of families. There are two genetic links—one involving problems on chromosome 14 and the other on chromosome 21—that tie into those families.

Otherwise, the genetic factor increases only about 8 percent for the child of a parent with Alzheimer's. Even if there are other members of your family with Alzheimer's, this does not prove there is any genetic factor.

As part of the research into the genetic factor, scientists have been trying to breed generations of mice that developed an Alzheimer-like disease, with some success. Their ultimate aim is to understand the genetic component, and then concurrently, to develop drugs which will intervene in the disease process.

Even if there is a genetic link, it does not prove you will have Alzheimer's, or even that you might. It only carries an extra risk factor. Try not to worry about this.

VIRUS

Some researchers are looking into the question of Alzheimer's relation to a slow virus, or to prions, which are even smaller than viruses. These studies are still inconclusive. However, there is no evidence that Alzheimer's disease is infectious or transmittable from person to person.

AUTOIMMUNE THEORY

One theory says that the mechanism of Alzheimer's disease is the breakdown of the body's natural defense system, the immune system, causing it to attack itself. Another says that the presence of toxins, genetic triggers or trauma, causes the immune system to be at war with itself.

Both these theories are based on the observation that people with Alzheimer's seem to have an abnormally low level of the proteins used to fight off infections. While investigations continue, there is no absolute confirmation of these theories yet.

DIETARY FACTORS

Some researchers are looking into the vitamin factor, especially the connection to B-complex deficiency. It is known that temporary dementia can be attributed to vitamin B deficiencies, and there are still many unanswered questions about whether Alzheimer's itself is also connected with dietary deficiencies.

HEAD INJURY

Studies have shown a greater prevalence of head injuries amongst people who later develop Alzheimer's disease, but the exact role is not at all clear.

APO E GENE TEST FOR DIAGNOSING ALZHEIMER'S

A new report issued in July, 1996, from the Duke University Medical School suggests that the apo E gene may hold clues, or even—according to researchers—the answer to detecting Alzheimer's disease.

All human beings are born with one of three variations of the apo E gene. University researchers found that those with the variation known as apo E-4 have been linked to a high risk of developing Alzheimer's disease as early as 60 to 70 years of age.

The research team carried out genetic testing on the tissues of 67 people who had been diagnosed with probable Alzheimer's disease (remembering that Alzheimer's disease is, so far, never a definite diagnosis). They found that 43 out of the 67 who had been diagnosed had the E-4 variant of the gene and that the brain autopsies backed up the diagnosis of Alzheimer's.

The results suggest that testing for apo E-4 in live patients may bring the detection of Alzheimer's disease from unsupported suppositions to confirmation. This would eradicate more expensive tests—such as imaging and CAT scans—and also make a diagnosis more sure. It would also enable patients to be identified for earlier treatment if such treatment existed.

However, as with all such reports, it is wise to be cautious before assuming that this is indeed the answer to the diagnosis. Although we may hope that this is indeed a definitive way to diagnose Alzheimer's, we should be aware of the inherent flaws of this very limited study. First, 14 of those tested did *not* have apo E-4 present in their genetic makeup, although the autopsies did confirm the presence of typical Alzheimer's brain degeneration. An additional 10 also did *not* have the apo E-4 and also did *not* show typical Alzhiemer's-like brain degeneration, although in life they had shown all the manifestations of dementia. This means that 43 people had the gene apo E-4 and an Alzheimer-like dementia, while 24 people had an Alzheimer-like dementia but no apo E-4 gene.

This suggests the possibilty that there is roughly a 65 percent chance of diagnosing Alzhiemer's accurately, *if*—and this a very big if—the apo E-4 gene turns out to be such an important indicator. However, until a sufficient number of healthy people in the same age group have been tested, the validity of the test is quite uncertain.

Considering that national statistics report about 10 percent of the population beween the ages of 60 to 70 years old have Alzheimer's disease, the apo E-4 gene might be found in 65 percent of that 10 percent. This means that slightly over half the people who are diagnosed with Alzheimer's disease also have the apo E-4 gene. But, it does not indicate that those who have the apo E-4 gene *will* or even *may* develop Alzheimer's.

Thus, we can only hope that this turns out to be a significant development, but we must not yet assume that it is. At this stage it is more of a pointer towards future hope.

As yet, all these questions remain just that, questions, to which we have no definite answers. We may find that numerous factors come together to cause the breakdown of the physical brain which we classify as Alzheimer's disease, and that we shall have to approach the question of treatments and cures on that basis, as a multifaceted campaign.

Much of the current research concentrates on interrupting the process of degeneration, since it is easier to document the actual physical degeneration than to figure out the causes. Therefore, a lot of research concentrates on developing brain chemicals to replace missing or depleted chemicals, and other drugs to promote functions which have been in decline.

However, this is a very volatile field and has been for 20 years. Because its cause is still unknown, new theories tend to come and go and then sometimes recur with confusing rapidity. Even the very basic things we think we know about Alzheimer's are still not established *beyond doubt.*

Here are some of the things we do not know. Despite the claims of Dr. Alzheimer and the additional research since the late 1960s, there are still a number of researchers questioning whether such a disease as Alzheimer's really exists.

Some of the most prominent brain cell researchers at Harvard have raised the question of whether what we call Alzheimer's disease is not, after all, merely the extreme edge of the aging arc. The problem is that we do not know enough about the aging body and the aging brain. We do know that all aging brains show signs of plaques and tangles. But, how many plaques and tangles are too many? Where is the dividing line between normal attrition and a disease process?

This is further complicated by the fact that brain degeneration and the actual dysfunction do not always correlate. People severely impaired in life have been found at autopsy to have only moderate brain degeneration, while others with severe brain degeneration were never diagnosed in life as having Alzheimer's disease. The official medical line is that Alzheimer's disease can only be truly established at autopsy, but even autopsy does not really supply that answer as clearly as we might hope.

You may have read in various reports that there are definitive tests which can be carried out to establish Alzheimer's disease. The presence of amyloid proteins, for example.

Unfortunately, the media does not always reveal the whole story. The first exciting news that people with Alzheimer's have abnormally large amounts of amyloid proteins in their cells and that this could lead to a simple skin test for Alzheimer's has not turned out to be true. Researchers have since found that healthy people, too, have amyloid proteins in their cells, although perhaps fewer. No such tests have developed.

It is very important not to let yourself be thrown into confusion by occasional sensational stories of tests, cures, and treatments. Be very cautious and know that you have not yet heard the whole story. Do some of your own research into the documentation. Usually, such stories are culled from academic papers, and you can track those down and use your common sense.

Do not go rushing all over the country or all over the world in pursuit of some touted cure or treatment. That is a fear reaction, not a hope reaction.

On the other hand, do not swallow the official line without question. The harsh fact is that the medical establishment has achieved very little in the last 20 years that has helped a single person with Alzheimer's disease or a single family. This is partly because it takes a long time to learn enough about a disease before finding treatments and cures. However, when so little is being offered, you are entitled to do some exploring of your own.

It is clear that dietary factors need further exploration. You can become a doctor in the United States without even studying nutrition in medical school, a frightening thought considering that food is our main source of health, and sometimes a serious part of ill-health.

Other areas of exploration such as homeopathy, herbs, Chinese herbal remedies, detoxification, counseling, therapy, bodywork, and exercise, may also supplement the life quality of a person with Alzheimer's. Unfortunately, families have been discouraged from trying any experimental interventions while being offered little or nothing in return, except experimental drugs with high toxicity problems.

This book assumes that you are intelligent enough to make your own choices and that you want to learn about any other possible lines of inquiry, with or without approval.

You are probably eager to know what exactly medical science is planning to offer you as a treatment or cure for Alzheimer's disease.

FUTURE TREATMENTS FOR ALZHEIMER'S

DRUGS

It is unlikely that one drug will be found that overcomes Alzheimer's disease, but researchers are looking at a variety of approaches to dealing with symptoms.

a) *Cognex* is currently being used in a national experimental program. This drug originally appeared on the market as THA (tetrahydroaminoacridine), or tacrine, and was said to help with memory loss problems. After a first burst of great enthusiasm, it was found that some of the alleged results were not as positive as publicity claimed, and a number of cases showed signs of severe liver problems as a result of using the drug. The FDA pulled it off the market.

However, outcry from families desperate for anything resulted in the reinstatement of the drug for experimental use, this time under the name Cognex. Those who take the drug have to be closely monitored for signs of liver damage, but families from around the country report a variety of responses to its use.

Some people report considerable improvement, while other report little or none. From anecdotal evidence, it seems to be most helpful in the earlier stages of Alzheimer's when memory problems can be improved with its use.

The drug is being heavily promoted at workshops and seminars by Cognex salesmen, and you should always keep the source of such information in mind. The manufacturer maintains a 1-800 hotline, but families report considerable pressure to maintain the drug, despite side effects.

Obviously, this is something worth trying, but it is also necessary to be cautious. It has not been established that Cognex does anything to cure or perhaps ultimately even to affect the long-term course of the disease.

b) *Desferrioxamine* is being used by some researchers to remove aluminum from the brain. Studies contradict one other on this whole issue so it remains open.

c) *Anti-beta amyloid drugs* are being developed to try to cut down on the over-production of beta amyloid protein found in people with Alzheimer's.

BRAIN CHEMICALS

Since a number of imbalances in brain chemicals have been noted, some researchers have been concentrating on synthesizing the missing chemicals and supplying them.

a) *Acetylcholine:* Low levels of acetylcholine acetyltransferase (CAT) mean that the chemical messenger system of the brain is afflicted. Therefore, the target of many laboratory researchers is to find the replacement for the missing chemical messengers.

b) *Lecithin* is one of the substances needed by the brain for the production of acetylcholine. It is found in many foods, and some researchers have been giving it to Alzheimer's patients. Results are disappointing so far, but some families report success with it.

c) *Choline* is another helper in the production of acetylcholine, and it is found in food. Researchers have fed it to people with Alzheimer's as an additive, but results are disappointing.

Despite the official line on lecithin and choline, individual families who have bought such substances from health food stores and given it to afflicted family members report some improvements. Therefore, it is important to carry out your own exploration, remembering never to exceed any recommended dosage.

FETAL BRAIN CELL TISSUE

This has not been explored in Alzheimer's at this point. Researchers have carried out transplants in a few cases of people with Parkinson's disease.

Some good results were found in one or two of the cases but not in others. Apart from the extremely experimental nature of the research, other people might well have issues with the ethics of using aborted fetuses in this way. Some think this may be the wave of the future for Alzheimer's.

GENETIC RESEARCH

So much false excitement is generated around genetic research, mainly because people greatly misunderstand its real potential. Also, we may yet find that *all* disease is associated with genetic factors. However, since at least two of the early-onset Alzheimer's are associated with gene defects, researchers are currently exploring this area.

NERVE GROWTH FACTORS

Brain cells are developed through nerve growth factors. While other nerve cells outside the central nervous system can regenerate, brain cells are not thought to be able to do this. However, researchers are looking for ways to stimulate the nerve growth factors to bring about renewed brain-cell development.

Every line of inquiry may well produce a treatment or even a cure. There is varied research being conducted, and families often find this very frustrating. Their natural desire is for a simple cause, followed by a simple treatment or cure. However, uncovering the mysteries of Alzheimer's is a very complex matter for it involves the most complicated organ in the body, the brain, an area which medical science still knows little about. It also involves examining the lives of long-lived people, which could include literally thousands of factors. Alzheimer's disease itself varies immensely varied from person to person. The research is vast, but, one day soon, we may very well read about that breakthrough from the huge amount of exploration, so never lose hope.

Family Crisis Alzheimer's Style

....

> *"Until my mother got Alzheimer's disease, I had five*
> *brothers and sisters. Now I might as well be an only child.*
> *I've been the one to look after her. I've been the one to make*
> *decisions about her. I'm the one who never gets a holiday.*
> *They're the ones with all the opinions—and they certainly*
> *had plenty of them when it came to selling her house so she*
> *could go into care. I can hardly bring myself to speak to them*
> *now and our mother's been dead for three years."*
>
> —PAULINE, age 47

Unfortunately, Pauline's story is not unusual. Alzheimer's disease, because it can go on for so long and because dealing with it is endlessly arguable, can pull families apart. It is a disease of function rather than of physical body, therefore it can cause endless dysfunction in the family itself. This is why it is very important for all family members to tackle the Alzheimer's problem together from the outset, if they can.

As families deal with life, so do they deal with disease. Given that Alzheimer's is a disruptive yet often subtle disease, infinitely variable, it tends to bring about family crisis, even in the best organized and healthiest of families. This is because the beginnings of the disease involve gradual loss of ability to function well in life, rather than specific symptoms needing specific treatment. It is a disease of behaviors, and families have to make decisions about their own behaviors in response to the illness. In families with unhealthy interaction patterns, Alzheimer's disease becomes a new battleground.

Even for healthy families, it brings many moments of crisis. There are a whole series of difficult decisions to be made, even though the family may lack sufficient information to make them. Often, they are working without support, without help and without any education in Alzheimer's disease and its ramifications.

The major crisis throughout is that family members are forced to revise their relationship with the person who is ill. A spouse has to adjust to loss of partnership while at the same time gradually taking on total care of someone who is beginning to function at primal levels, like a child. A son or daughter must face the gradual loss of a parent. It is hard for any child to take on a parental role toward a parent. To do so goes against family history with its psychic life and all the complications of parent-child relationships. Moreover, Alzheimer's brings additional fears to the children of its victims, as they wonder if this is a picture of their own future. It is a meeting place of loss, fear, and yearning.

Since we know that many families in the United States today are tied to unhealthy patterns of relating, we can expect to find them entangled in the Alzheimer world too. There the care of the sick person becomes a desperately embattled business. Siblings are likely to find all their old issues revive, with unanswered needs and suppressed angers coming to the surface. A child who has seldom received nurturing care from a parent will find it harder than most people to become that parent's caregiver. Family members who have not learned to respect and cherish each other are not likely to treat the sick person with respect, appropriate attention, and acceptance. The unhealthy rivalries and wars arise again, all fought out in the shadow of one of the most demanding of illnesses.

These battles can be subtle. Merely because your family is not actually fighting does not mean you have escaped dysfunctional patterns. The following are among the signs of unhealthy family attitudes around Alzheimer's:

Denial. Family members deny to each other that the situation is as serious as it really is, often treating the afflicted person as if he or she could choose to manage better. The sick family member is blamed for not trying hard enough, being too needy, or deliberately behaving badly when showing symptoms of the disease. Family members may come up with a list of elaborate explanations that deny the existence of the illness. One family, for example, talked about "Mother's nerves," not her Alzheimer's disease.

The family may deride or castigate the sick family member for exhibiting the symptoms of illness. "Ma, I told you that already!"—as if the person did not have memory problems. "She doesn't even wash properly any more—it's disgusting!"—as if the sick person is being deliberately offensive.

Anger. Family members become enraged with each other over differing opinions on treatment, plans for the sick person, or each other's behavior. They are unable to let go of their demands on each other or forgive each other's shortcomings in coping with the illness. Sometimes this rage is directed at the person who is sick, either as obvious abuse or more subtly as constant criticism, irritation, and demeaning treatment. "Look, Mom, you've got to stop phoning me any time you want some little thing done. You've got to be more independent," says a son to his mother who is being overwhelmed by her illness and finding it impossible to function in daily life without help.

Despair. A constant mood of depression and frustration may combine with grief to the point of feeling completely hopeless. Says one spouse, "Every morning when I wake up, I remember Hal's sick and then I just think, oh, let me lie here, don't let the day even start."

While it is natural for any one to have a grief reaction to learning that a family member has Alzheimer's disease, if the feeling deepens into lingering despair, this is an unhealthy response. It is true that there is no effective treatment for Alzheimer's right now, neither is there a cure. However, there are still ways to make life feel worthwhile and emotionally valuable, even in the midst of the crisis of living with an incurable illness.

We have seen many people begin to deal with this situation— people with cancer, people with AIDS—and it is time for people with Alzheimer's, and their caregivers, to begin to find the best ways of dealing with this disease. Alzheimer's is a disease lived both by the person who has it and by the caregiver. When the caregiver sinks into despair, as much as we may sympathize, the situation is not being dealt with.

Caregivers must be encouraged to seek healthy coping patterns, not sanctioned to give way to unhealthy patterns. Despair is an unhealthy pattern.

Blame. The blaming family is only too commonly found in the Alzheimer world. Instead of uniting to form a battle strategy to deal with the disease, working out family approaches and coming to consensus, the family breaks apart. This division tends to continue for years after the crisis, separating siblings and other relatives. It happens both because there has previously been a pattern of divisiveness but also, because of the family's inability to face loss, fear, and the pressures of role change. Family members blame each other instead of confronting their own feelings about the disease.

Avoidance. We see this in family members refusing to talk about the disease with the person who has it—"I couldn't possibly tell my husband he has Alzheimer's. It would really upset him and I don't want to hurt him."

This may sound like consideration but it is actually the speaker's inability to reach out to the other in a painful situation. It echoes the old habit of secrecy around cancer and it condemns the real victim—the person with Alzheimer's—to loneliness and fear. The person who has the disease has invariably known for years something awful was wrong. Others do that person no favor when they deny the opportunity to speak about what is happening. Often, bizarre behaviors are triggered by family refusal to break the silence around Alzheimer's.

One man asked his support group just when they thought he should tell his wife she had Alzheimer's. "She begs me to tell her what's wrong with her and why she keeps forgetting everything," he explained, "but I don't want to upset her."

The support group facilitator explained gently that by her question his wife was giving him permission to tell her. This often happens. The person who has the illness comments on being stupid, being worthless, being crazy, mentions that something is wrong, talks about memory problems. All these are clues that suggest it is time to talk about Alzheimer's.

When someone says, "I forget so much," it is not a kindness to gloss it over by saying, "Oh well, we all forget things. I'm always forgetting things myself." It is better to show understanding and empathy by saying something like, "It must be hard to forget such a lot, but it's not your fault, you know. You have an illness that causes you to forget things." Usually, people are surprisingly accepting of such news, even relieved by it.

For those who are strongly attached to the need for denial, there will still be denial, "What? Are you crazy or something?" one man retorted when his wife tried to tell him he was ill. On that and many other occasions, he accused her of being the crazy one. This was a clear message from him that he was not ready to admit the truth. Since he had always been a dominating and selfish man, this simply meant he was not about to give up control to anyone else at that point, illness or no illness. Nothing will shake a denier, so family members need not worry that the truth will hurt them. They will brush it off.

Another often hurtful example of avoidance is when family members do not come to visit the person who has Alzheimer's. Either they reduce all contacts to occasional short drop-ins, or they call from time to time on the telephone. If the person is moved into a full-time care facility, they seldom visit. When they do visit, they are reluctant to sit down and take time to listen to or be with the person. Often certain family members exhibit such avoidance while others carry all the caregiving burden. Such behavior may designate selfishness or emotional immaturity in being unwilling to deal with the reality of the issue, or it may indicate serious emotional maladjustment to all the issues of old age, disease, death, and loss.

"My sister never comes to see Mother. She says it's too painful. Well, I say too bad for her. Who's supposed to do the coping—nobody? Doesn't she think it's painful for me? But I'm here doing it," says one embittered caregiver, who says she will not forgive her sister.

"We're five brothers and sisters, and four of us are closely involved with looking after our dad. Our oldest brother keeps away, but he sends money when we need it. Well, we figure that's just his way. We know he can't manage to be here. I don't know how it'll be for him later—knowing he wasn't here when we needed him—but at least we all feel we're doing everything we can," says a caregiver from a different family.

These differences in commitment certainly divide families, but the caregivers who do the best in their resolution of the Alzheimer's journey are those who forgive the failings of others. They are the people wise enough to know that they will lose something valuable from their own lives by holding onto grudges and resentments and angers.

A common form of avoidance occurs once the person becomes more deeply impaired and is not able to initiate communication or be cognitively accurate. Family members say, "I won't go and see Grandma any more. There's no point. She doesn't know me."

This raises the question of whether seeing Grandma is for the family member's benefit or Grandma's. It does not answer the other question of who will love Grandma if the family doesn't. We all need love and caring and we all feel better when we get it. People who work in care homes report commonly that someone who gets good family attention shows the emotional difference. It is hard to say cognitively what the difference is, but the person is fuller, enriched, less anxious, less yearning when a loving family visit has occurred.

There is never a time when love is irrelevant. Grandma always needs love. Love does not mean an exchange of historically accurate data with names, faces, and times correct. Love means being patient, being attentive, holding Grandma's hand, and maybe doing nothing but being loving. It is a pity that families so often withdraw their attention when Grandma can no longer pass the biodata test. Even people in comas are now known to be responsive to stimulus, conversation, and people holding their hands. People with Alzheimer's are far more conscious than people in comas. They are present. They need present love.

The family that avoids visits is avoiding in the short term its feelings of pain, loss, and helplessness, but all of these feelings tend to catch up in the long run. Guilt over unfulfilled duties and omissions of love lasts a lifetime and often creates the dread of being similarly abandoned in need or old age. If we demonstrate that our elderly are not valued, we set our-selves in time to also be valueless to our family members. If we show that love and caring are always valuable, we teach our children something worthwhile about loving.

THE DESIGNATED CAREGIVER SYNDROME

Sometimes there may be only one family member to care for the sick person, but more often the family quietly designates one member to do the caregiving. There is no pattern to this designation. Sometimes it will be an unmarried daughter, more rarely an unmarried son, but it may also be one particular family member whether married or not, with children or not. This obviously connects with previously assumed family roles. Perhaps that person volunteered in the past to carry out caregiver roles. Perhaps that person has merely not resisted being put into the role.

However the selection takes place, the designated caregiver often is left to do all the caregiving without any practical family help other than long-distance telephone calls offering opinions, advice, and criticism. The caregiver becomes virtually deserted by the rest of the family except when major decisions are involved. Even then, they may not get support from the family but only input. It is not only siblings who elect a designated caregiver. Children do it to parents too.

"I look after my wife all the time and I love her very much. I'd never put her away anywhere," relates one caregiver. "But I hardly ever get to sleep through the night any more and it's real hard to take care of the house. I got two daughters but they're pretty busy so I thought maybe I should get a woman in to help so I could get a little break. My daughters say, 'Oh Daddy, don't,' so I didn't."

His daughters, however, didn't help any more than before, so the father was left alone to cope with his increasingly impaired wife. He felt that he could not risk losing the emotional approval of his daughters and therefore he was trapped as the designated caregiver.

Another way designated caregivers become trapped is when geographically distant family members deny the extent of the ill-ness. This often happens because of the sick person's ability to cover up and put on a good social front in a telephone conversation. If those family members never come to visit, they have no means of checking out their perception of the situation. It is not uncommon for them to suggest that the caregiver is exaggerating the problems.

There are a number of ways in which the designated caregivers can prevent themselves being caught in this way, although it may be emotionally hard for them to do so. For distant relatives who do not understand the situation, there is an easy solution. Insist that they come to relieve you of duty for a weekend or a week. If proving a point is your aim, a weekend will usually do it. One weekend spent with a person who has Alzheimer's disease is like boot camp, a thorough basic training in what the caregiver's life is really like. This has set many a family straight and ensured that at least they do not emotionally sabotage the work being done by denying the seriousness of the situation.

The designated caregiver must set limits, as hard as this can be. Family members must be asked for definite times and commitments to allow the caregiver time off. The designated caregiver must not give way on this, but should tough it out. If family members are geographically close, ask them for a weekly break, at least. If they are far away, then yearly or twice-yearly relief is not unreasonable. If children resist helping, then hire the help you need. If your money is short, ask the children to help pay for hired help.

The designated caregiver must also do as much outreach as possible into the community for additional help. All possible day respite programs should be used (see "Day Centers" in Chapter 9). Friends should be asked for occasional help. Hiring a few hours of help a week should definitely be considered. You will find a wider range of suggestions throughout this book. Use them all.

FAMILY COUNCIL SESSIONS

Unless your family is dysfunctional in a major way, it may be hard to recognize that you are actually dealing with dysfunction. If, however, you find that a number of the patterns outlined here are present in your family, take steps to deal with the problem. If the family is not suffering from major permanent patterns of dysfunction, you will be able to bring positive approaches to the situation.

Try the family council as a way of coping, perhaps with the help of an Alzheimer's care professional. It is often easier for outsiders to bring up subjects that family members may tacitly help each other avoid.

When families resolve to deal with the situation together rather than struggling in self-destructive warfare, they can effectively meet the crisis of Alzheimer's.

The following suggestions outline a way for the family to begin a campaign of coping with this crisis. This can then become a process of developing and maintaining a family plan to meet the needs of the person with Alzheimer's. There are many ways to do this, and the suggested method is merely one that you and your family could use. It has a number of components that take your family through the planning process. This plan allows family members freedom to be honest, limits tendencies to criticize or interfere with each other, and follows practical lines along which you can all plan your Alzheimer campaign.

It is necessary for family members to agree to abide by the rules outlined here. If you anticipate severe problems with compliance, you might find it useful to call in an outsider who will act as the mediator for your meeting. You may also pick one family member to play this role or simply use the outline in this book as your facilitator, reminding each other of the rules when appropriate.

The biggest problem will be time limitations. This plan suggests very short time limits. Some families may insist on longer ones. In fact, you can take as long as your family wishes, provided everyone agrees. You can increase the times suggested here by any ratio your family needs. However, experience shows that strict time limits bring about clear planning. Adapt these guidelines to your needs. If you want to take an entire weekend for this council session, it will not be time wasted.

THE FAMILY COUNCIL PROCEDURE

The first requirement for the family council is that everyone agrees to be bound by rules and decisions. The rules include time limits for each person to speak. Each member agrees to allow the others to say their piece without interruption, correction, argument, or reproach. This allows each person to speak freely but within the agreed time. You must all agree to the following limits:

- Do not attack each other.
- Do not bring up the past.
- Do not speculate about each other's future behavior.
- Respect each other's differences.
- Agree to abide by planning decisions on a consensus basis, which might mean that not everyone agrees in detail with everything. You all must become open to compromise in order to implement an effective plan.

FIRST STEP:
PERSONAL ALZHEIMER'S STATEMENTS

Each person has five minutes (or some other time limit) to speak without interruption and answer the following question: *What is your hope and what is your personal need in this situation?*

Some people might prefer to think it over and make notes for their answer.

Here is an example of how a family answered this question. They were four children who had met together to discuss how to deal with the fact that their widowed mother had been diagnosed with Alzheimer's disease and was not doing well living at home alone. She had been a difficult mother for all of them, angry and often critical.

TED

I really hope that Mother can stay in her own home as long as possible. I don't want her to go into some nursing home and be unhappy there or get treated badly. On the other hand, I know I don't want to look after her. She's never shown any respect for who I am or what I want, and I can't deal with that. I guess I kind of love her deep down, but frankly most of the time I'm with her, I just feel really mad at her. I know I'd be bad at looking after her.

SUE

I want Mom to be well looked after. I don't think she's doing well at home and I'm certainly not moving back in with her. I couldn't wait to leave home and I'm not about to let go of my own life at this point. I need my space. I won't give it up for her. I still find her really hard to deal with, and she gets worse the sicker she gets.

BILL

I'd like Mother to stay in her own home. I know she wants that. I'll bet we can get someone good to stay with her. I don't mind coming over sometimes and staying. I don't pay any attention to her being critical. It's just her way. It doesn't mean anything. I need to know I did my best for her, and I don't mind putting some of my own life aside to help her now. That's okay with me.

ANN

I don't honestly know what I feel about our mother. I wish it was her who'd died and our father who was still alive. I'd have been prepared to have him live with us in our home but not her. She'd break up my marriage if I let her over the threshold and I want this marriage to work. I don't even know if I could help look after her at all. Since Fred and I are pretty comfortably off, we could help financially with whatever we decide to do, but I want to keep physically as much out of this as I can.

Plainly, these family members want very different things, have very different relationships with their mother, and would probably each come to a different conclusion about what to do. However, it is still possible for them to reach a consensus that may not be anyone's best individual plan. The most important thing about the hope and need statement is that it really is honest and that family members do not reproach each other or try to persuade each other to feel differently. It may seem hard to accept that some children do not love or even necessarily like their parent, but that is the reality. It is necessary to recognize this without criticism. The abuse, mistreatment, and abandonment of aged parents comes when feelings are not being dealt with honestly.

SECOND STEP:
WHAT IS YOUR GREATEST DIFFICULTY?

Each family member should take three minutes to outline his or her greatest difficulty in dealing with the situation. Typically the greatest difficulties involve unresolved feelings about the person—"I always hated him"—or feelings about Alzheimer's itself.

"I'm scared I'm going to get this disease too," says Ted. "I look at Mom and I wonder if that's going to be me in thirty years. I'm kind of disgusted when I see what's happening. You know, she doesn't dress nicely any more. The house is dirty. At least I always used to respect her, even if I didn't always like her. It's hard to admit I'm judging her for being ill, but I guess I am."

THIRD STEP:
WHAT ARE THE GREATEST NEEDS HERE?

Family members should make a list of what they see as the most important problems to be dealt with. This could be done in five minutes; conversation about the list should be kept to the minimum. A needs list might include the following:

1. help in the house

2. daily visits from family members

3. financial supervision

4. shopping, laundry, cooking

5. coping with loneliness and social isolation

6. coping with fear, suspicion, anxiety

The lists will vary. The person may need total help or occasional input. Each family member will have noticed different things that require attention, and comparing lists will help them develop a total picture of what is going on. The discussion will also include decisions about what are immediate needs and what can be reviewed again in the near future.

FOURTH STEP:
MAKING THE FAMILY PLAN

This section is one that requires discussion, perhaps a lot of it. Family members should keep in mind that they need to reach a consensus, for which compromise is necessary.

Divide the plan into immediate action and future action. Under immediate action, you might suggest all the things that could be done to enable the person to stay at home, if family members agree to this. It is usual for the ultimate plan to change according to the development of the illness. It may be possible to keep the person at home with various kinds of support and intervention, then later perhaps to bring someone into the home, then to consider a small home residence placement, and ultimately perhaps to consider a nursing home.

FIFTH STEP:
MAKING COMMITMENTS

This is very important because differing personal commitments cause problems. The purpose of this step is to decide how to act on the needs list, either to make sure each identified need is taken care of or, in some cases, to agree to put off certain decisions until a later date. The checklist of needs is your focus for individual commitment, but family members may also commit to other actions that are not on the list, such as agreeing to make social visits three times a week.

Each individual must state honestly what his or her personal commitment is in time, in money, and in actions. That statement has to be accepted by everyone present. This will touch on all the inequalities of the family situation. One sister lives far away so she cannot give daily, weekly, or even monthly time. Neither does she have much money, so she cannot help financially. However, there may be other ways she can contribute. Perhaps a richer sibling can pay her way to take care of Mother for two weeks a year while someone else gets time off from caregiving. Perhaps she could telephone Mother every evening for a short conversation and another sibling could pick up the bill. Together, the family can think of a number of ways of helping each other to contribute. All such offers must be based on each member's expressed wish to do something, not on pressure family members place on each other.

This is not the place to say, "Oh yeah, Ted, you always say you'll do stuff and then you never follow through." If Ted makes a commitment and later does not stand by it, that is material for the next family council. Ted's possible future behavior is not up for discussion in this meeting. Family members have to accept each other's commitment. They must not expect one member to do more work than the others merely because that person lives nearer Mother.

The family needs to work out some kind of equity based on voluntary commitment. It will not work for three members to say, "Well, Ted, we're all doing so much. How come you're not?" Each person has to commit himself, not try to railroad someone else into an equal workload.

It is hard for family members to sit by while one of them simply does not make as big a donation of time, money, or effort. However, the point of this family council is to ensure that the needs of the person with Alzheimer's are met. It is not the purpose of this meeting to make sure everyone is contributing equally. That may be the hope of the meeting, but it is not its focus.

It is hard for families to let go of their expectations of each other. It does indeed violate basic feelings about fairness when one person does a lot more than another. For that matter, it is unfair. However, being fair is not the purpose of this meeting. Carrying out an effective care plan is the purpose.

Neither is this meeting for replaying old family resentments, angers, disappointments, and feuds. This is why the guidelines suggest so many limits on time and allowing each person uninterrupted speech without comment. As hard as that may be, it is a healthy way to work through a crisis. Perhaps it will introduce some helpful new patterns of relating within the family.

A good positive way to close this meeting is for each member to write down one or more ways in which he or she will support the others in carrying out the care plan for the person with Alzheimer's. Family members might agree to make regular telephone calls to each other. Sister Sue might offer to take Ann's children to school the morning after Ann has done her regular overnight sleepover at Mother's. Ted might offer to foot the bill for certain items, and so on.

It is also an extra gift for each family member to write one positive thing they appreciate about each person present and then to read it out loud. Although this may sound too touchy-feely for some people, the sad fact is that family members hardly ever tell each other what they appreciate, admire, or enjoy about each other. They assume others know they love them when this is often far from the truth. It never ever hurts to tell what you appreciate about an individual.

To summarize the family council plan:

1. Agree to time limits, no interruptions, no criticisms. Keep focused on making a plan to meet the needs of the person with Alzheimer's.

2. Start with a hope-and-need statement, written (5 minutes) and/or spoken (5 minutes).

3. Make a greatest-difficulty statement, with reference to the person and/or the disease (3 minutes).

4. Make a greatest-needs list in order of urgency, first as individuals and then coming to consensus on a family list (5 minutes for the first, 10 minutes for the family list).

5. Discuss the family plan for immediate action, based upon the needs list and perhaps on other issues of care raised in this discussion (allow 20 minutes or more if needed, but be disciplined about keeping it on track).

6. Make invidual commitment statements, in which each person commits to what he or she will do or take responsibility for (2 minutes).

7. Make support statements and individual appreciation statements (2 minutes per person).

At the end of the first family meeting, a date and time should be set for the next meeting. In the meantime all family members should agree to educate themselves as much as possible about the Alzheimer journey and their own pathways as Alzheimer companions.

Some families feel the council plan would not work for them. One man said, "I know my family and they don't like the idea of being restricted in their time requirements. Does this really work?"

The answer is: It works as well as any council meetings. That means there is a basic formula for conducting the meeting from which people will constantly divert. Like your own local city or town council, as long as the actual business of the meeting is fulfilled, the time and the individual discussions can vary widely.

The real answer is that, yes, family councils work, if family members make them work. One family of four adult children made such a plan for the care of their mother. They came to her home for their discussion. It took a weekend. They often diverted from the plan but they achieved consensus. They designated an on-the-spot daughter as official caregiver, and all agreed to abide by her decisions. Two others gave monetary support and general encouragement. The other daughter, about to embark on a sailing trip around the world, telephoned in from every port of call.

In their plan they also agreed to use their mother's income and savings to pay for whatever extra caregivers were needed in order to keep their mother at home until she died. In fact, she did die peacefully at home.

In another family, two sisters and a niece flew from the East Coast to meet in California with a brother and an uncle to have a family council on their mother's fate. This family also used the family council guidelines, and the majority of the members were able to come to agreement, although the brother could not accept his mother's Alzheimer's and therefore remained peripheral in her care. This continued an emotional division that had previously existed in the family.

Like any plan, the family council works if people agree to make it work.

Education and Acceptance—
The Secret of Alzheimer's Success

"No one tells you what to do for the best. Doctors don't seem to know. Leastways, ours sure didn't. People like us don't know about this thing and it's real hard to find out. I was lucky, I guess. My neighbor went through all this with his wife. When I moved in with my mother, he was real helpful to me. I sort of followed along in his footsteps. But I never felt real sure of doing right by her."

—PAUL, 45, whose mother had Alzheimer's disease but died of a stroke

M any people start out like Paul, not knowing what to do. Too many people end up the same way. It can be hard to find the right information about Alzheimer's disease. The biggest problem is that the help most people need is not available from medical sources, on the whole. What most people need to know is how to live with Alzheimer's, what to expect and how to deal with the problems peculiar to this illness. Most of these problems are not really medical. Many of them are behavioral. Many of the solutions are also behavioral in that they ask changes of the family of the person with Alzheimer's.

Until people understand two things, they are in constant trouble. One is that Alzheimer's demands behavior changes of everyone living with the disease—everyone, that is, except the person who has it. Two, everyone lives with Alzheimer's disease in his or her own way.

The biggest single problem families have is that they do not accept these two truths. They fight, deny, or ignore the changes that they must undergo, and they lock themselves into an unwinnable battle by demanding that the person with Alzheimer's change, adapt, or somehow get retrained. So the greatest part of the family's education must begin with education about the person who has the disease.

If you are a family caregiver, you are already an expert in this area. You know the person you are dealing with. You know what upsets that person, what pleases and what enrages. You know what that person can do. You know that sometimes, even though you do not understand why, that person's capacity to manage is greatly reduced. You probably know how to bribe, persuade, and cajole successfully to get your way most of the time. So you are already an expert in one area of Alzheimer's. Your first piece of education is to acknowledge that you are an expert. No doctor, nurse, or social worker knows your person like you do.

You might try noting down the things that you know about dealing with Alzheimer's. In fact, it would be educational for you to keep a daily journal. It will help you to get a grip on things and it will be a valuable record. If other people become involved in caring for the person with Alzheimer's, your journal will help them to know what works, what usually happens in certain situations, and how to deal with events. Such a journal need not be elaborate. You do not have to be a writer. Just jot things down. You will probably become aware of many more things as you do this.

It is also useful to learn as much as you can about the disease itself. In one way, this will not be easy since you probably already know more than most people. It is also true that we have very little real incontrovertible information available on this disease. You can learn about its typical behaviors, however, and this knowledge will help you and your family avoid battles you cannot win.

Although each person with Alzheimer's exhibits the illness in a very individual way, there are some general guidelines you can learn. One is that the symptoms of Alzheimer's can vary literally from day to day, usually according to the general condition of the person.

"I don't understand my mother," says Tom in despair. "One day she's fine. She can dress herself and put all her clothes on properly. That's normal for her, right? Then suddenly another day she can't do any of those things. I tell her to put her trousers on and she lays them on top of her thighs. She sticks her blouse on upside-down. I mean, what's going on?"

Probably what is going on is that Tom's mother is less well on her days of coping badly. This doesn't mean less well with Alzheimer's disease. She may have a cold or a touch of flu, a gastrointestinal problem, or maybe some emotional upset has happened. Any disturbance of health or emotional well-being can disrupt the Alzheimer patient's ability to function. In fact, ill health may show up only in increased malfunction.

In order to really learn from the person you are looking after, you need to be able to step back sometimes and be an impartial observer. That is not always easy, specially if you are angry or overtired. However, you will be better able to deal with the problems of caregiving if you can keep your role as observer. The biggest source of aggravation for a caregiver is the feeling that the person with Alzheimer's is deliberately doing things, or not doing them, to annoy, manipulate, or punish. Actually, each of these intentions would require the kind of rational ability to think things through that people with Alzheimer's specifically do not have.

To be the impartial observer, you need to be educated about who you are as a caregiver—especially about your emotional fragilities and your personal stress reactions. Again, a journal will help you to learn about yourself as a caregiver and enable you to watch out for the ways in that you can be caught up in the stress of the situation. There is no need to blame yourself. We are all human and as caregivers we all have our shortcomings, especially when we are tired or upset. But just to know yourself will help you make the appropriate allowances, for yourself and for the person you look after.

As part of your education about this disease, read the problem-solving section of Chapter 7, which will cover many of the intricacies of dealing with Alzheimer's that often only caregivers know about. Another way to learn more is to attend as many workshops, training classes, and seminars as you can find.

There is, unfortunately, a dearth of practical knowledge being given out in workshops. Too many of them deal with new medical research and the latest drug-testing experiments, subjects that do not relieve families where they most need relief. But go anyway and be prepared to ask questions. If you have particular requests, make a note of them before the workshop or seminar so that you will not forget them or be too intimidated to ask. Contact your local branch of the Alzheimer's Association and find out where support groups meet (see the Appendix).

Support groups are an important source of information for you. Caregivers know who the good doctors are, ways of dealing with problems, and the area's resources. They also know all the daily grind and its hardships, in a way that only caregivers can. It can bring you relief and a sense of peace just to be with people who know this situation.

Other parts of your education will include research into financial and legal issues. A husband and wife with shared resources need to look into safeguarding their assets, ensuring that power of attorney is taken care of, and doing their estate planning for the future. Unfortunately, until the health care system in this country is revised considerably, Alzheimer's disease can bankrupt a family. Forward-looking planning of the right kind can help to alleviate some of the financial burden. In the past, some couples have divorced simply so that they could protect their assets when one of them needed full-time placement in a nursing facility.

There are now a number of ways around such situations, but it is a highly specialized area with legalities and financial details varying considerably from state to state. Therefore, it is very important that you see an expert in this field. Usually that will be a lawyer with expertise and experience in elder law and elder estate planning, with special reference to issues of providing for long-term health care. Be sure the person you see really is an expert in these issues. Check out references and recommendations from local organizations—for example, the American Association of Retired Persons (AARP), your local Agency on Aging, elder services agencies, and senior centers. When you do find someone who is recommended, do not be shy about asking what experience that person has had in such estate planning. You want someone who has dealt with hundreds of clients needing such a service, not a handful. Be ruthless about your questions, because this professional can make or mar your own future financial well-being. Many experts suggest that you do not allow this person to also handle investing your finances.

If your family member has not yet had a diagnosis of Alzheimer's, that person might still be eligible for long-term care insurance. You obviously cannot get such insurance after the diagnosis, but you might get it before any suspicions you have about your family member are actually confirmed.

Be extremely careful about any such insurance and seek guidance from an independent advisor. Do not take out policies on the advice of your insurance agent alone. Take time to think things over and have the policy looked at by an independent expert. Ordinary health insurance will cover normal hospitalization even if Medicare does not, and few other policies cover long-term care although many claim to do so. The national headquarters of AARP reports that there are many spurious long-term care insurance policies around that, when the crunch comes, avoid paying out just when you need them to. Alzheimer's disease is covered by very few policies, so be suspicious and do not let yourself be talked into anything. Your local senior centers, senior services agencies, and AARP branches can probably help you with this matter.

If you are facing possible future placement of a family member, do not assume that you need either to have long-term care insurance or to pay out your own cash down to the verge of ruin. It is not true that you cannot keep your family member on in a care facility in which he or she is already comfortable after resources have been spent to the level at which and Medicaid takes over. Many reputable care facilities are part of a federal aid program that allows them to keep a resident on after the patient no longer has full financial resources. Such facilities get federal grants in return for being part of the program. You can get this information in advance and choose your facility accordingly, picking one that guarantees keeping your relative on once Medicaid kicks in.

Do not imagine that residents on Medicaid are treated any differently from those who are still paying full rates. They are not. State regulations these days ensure that every resident is treated with the same respect and gets the same care and attention. If this were not so, the institution could lose its license. Remember that money does not buy certainty when it comes to good care, so do not be too attached to having to pay for everything yourself.

As part of your education for the future, learn about the range of care facilities in your part of the world. Read Chapter 11 on placing someone in care so that you know well ahead of time what your alternatives are. Not everyone with advanced Alzheimer's disease has to be placed in a skilled nursing facility. Look around at small home care residences so that you have a good idea of other choices well ahead of making any. That way, you will not be caught by surprise or rushed into a decision you may regret.

Learn about the possible course of this disease, while also acknowledging that it can vary greatly. That way, you will recognize certain changes as they happen. For example, you will notice when vision changes cause a person to be unable to center on a chair or toilet seat and be ready to help act as a guide. You will be alerted then that you should probably be around your relative when he or she goes up and down stairs, just to keep an eye on safety hazards.

Knowing what is happening in the disease course will help you be much more accepting. For example, when you begin to realize that your relative is no longer connecting words with their meaning, you will not get angry when your questions or commands are not carried through.

"I told Miriam to switch off the light before she left the room. She nodded but she didn't do it. I told her six more times before I got mad at her and just went in and did it myself," says Paul, still angry as he tells the story. He will not win such battles because he is fighting against a fact of the disease—Miriam no longer knows what Paul is saying when he uses nouns whose meanings are lost to her. If he pointed to the objects represented by the nouns, she might get the meaning.

Such education keeps you sane. Another good way to keep sane is by educating yourself about good caregiving and about caring for yourself as a caregiver. This is very important. The biggest problem for caregivers is the drop in their own health due to lack of stress management. Read Chapter 10 on being a good caregiver and caring for yourself. This is often the most-neglected aspect of caregiving. Caregivers put themselves last, but unfortunately that only guarantees that they will not be effective in their task.

Make sure you go to any stress management classes you can find. Often, such classes are offered at senior centers, in recognition of the fact that life in old age can have many stresses. Do not dismiss these classes as if you could not learn anything useful. Take exercise classes, especially gentle exercises like yoga and tai chi. Learn about your diet and what it should consist of as you age. All of these things will be part of your education for survival.

Other ways of educating yourself could include learning how to communicate better, especially if your relationships with your family members are not going well. If you are an elder yourself, you might have learned ways of communicating (or not communicating) that do not serve you well any more. Relearning such habits and finding better ways to do things and talk about things will form part of your network of help. Basically, people only know what you tell them, and sometimes you have to learn how to be specific. You may need to brush up your habits of communication.

If you are caring for a member of your family, it is likely that you will be involved in that person's death process. If you know nothing about the process of death and dying, consider attending workshops or training courses on the subject. If there are no such workshops near you, or you just cannot bring yourself to attend them, there are very helpful books available. They are listed in the Bibliography at the back of this book. Read ahead of time so that you can become aware of how you feel about death and dying.

Be open to learning from experts how to cope better with life. Life with Alzheimer's has many burdens so do not scorn getting help, guidance, or a chance to talk things over with a counselor, therapist, or psychologist. Do not think that only people who are crazy would seek such help. It is common now for people to seek counseling when they are dealing with difficult situations. Talking things over with a professional can help you to see a situation more clearly. In the old days, family members were around more and could talk things over. Now many people do not even have a minister, priest, or rabbi to discuss life difficulties with, yet life has become incredibly complex. So allow yourself to get that extra help and input where it can do most good.

How can you determine whether a counselor could help? Take a look at this list:

1. I feel trapped and helpless.

2. I am tense and unhappy every day.

3. I can't face the day when I wake up.

4. I can't sleep.

5. I feel so guilty every time I get angry.

6. I don't know who to turn to.

7. I don't think I can go on much longer.

If any of these statements describe you, you could undoubtedly get help from counseling. To find a good counselor, ask your local senior services agency. Ask your doctor for references. Check out any local counseling offices or services. They are usually listed in the Yellow Pages under Counseling or Therapy. It may take one or two attempts to find the person you feel most comfortable with, but you will benefit from counseling. How many times you go is up to you. You will work it out with your therapist. Counseling does not have to be long-term or even very expensive. You will probably find that your health insurance covers at least part of the payment.

You must also educate yourself about the effect of medications on your relative. Once a person is manifesting Alzheimer's disease, the norms for body response change, becoming highly variable and individual. Drugs are never tested on people with dementias, except in the case of specific drugs for Alzheimer's.

This means that no one can say how a particular drug will affect a person who has Alzheimer's disease. The side effects that might be minor in reasonably healthy people can be devastating in Alzheimer's patient.

You must do two things to safeguard your relative. First, ask your doctor what the side effects of any new medication are, according to the manufacturer. If your doctor does not know, or seems to be shrugging you off with vague reassurances, ask the physician to give you the printed information on side effects provided by the manufacturer. This way, you know what to look out for. This is very important since your relative probably will not be able to tell you, "Oh I feel sick," or "My vision has gone blurry." You will have to watch for unusual behavior from your relative.

Keep daily notes after any change of medication so that you have a documentation of new behaviors or troubling developments. Do not accept the doctor's assurances that they are not due to the medication. Ask your doctor to test by withdrawing the medication to see whether behavior becomes normal again.

The second thing to do to safeguard your relative is to demand a change, reduction, or cessation of medication if drastic changes occur. Here is a family anecdote with a message. Albert had severe Alzheimer's disease and was regularly becoming very agitated at night. His wife, Sybil, mentioned this to his neurologist who then prescribed Haldol, a frequently prescribed medication in cases of Alzheimer agitation. If Sybil had asked the neurologist what the side effects of Haldol are, she would have learned that among them are confusion, memory loss, and tendency to falling. (You might think therefore that Haldol would not necessarily be the best choice for an Alzheimer patient, but that is another story.)

Albert became even more agitated, and the neurologist doubled the dose. He became more agitated again, and the neurologist increased the dose once more. Albert became violent and unmanageable, and his wife committed him to a nursing home Alzheimer unit. There, Albert's medication was immediately reduced and gradually tapered off altogether within the next three weeks. Albert never at any time became violent or even agitated. From this, his new doctor at the nursing home concluded that Albert was actually allergic to Haldol.

If Sybil had been better informed and aggresive in determining what was going on, possibly she need never have put Albert into care. The lesson here is to be demanding and to insist upon the validity of what you observe. You are not, unless you are a doctor, an expert on medications, but you are an expert on what is the usual behavior of your relative. You do not have to accept disadvantageous conditions that come about through medications. Since extremely little is known about the effects of medication on people with Alzheimer's, you are the resident expert on its effects upon your relative. Keep notes and be firm.

This brings us to the conclusion of the education campaign, that is intended merely to reinforce something that you may not have realized: you are the expert. You are the one who really knows the person with Alzheimer's. Even if you do not always know the best solutions for your problems, you are still the resident expert.

Dealing with Alzheimer's disease is such a divisive process that it seems appropriate to look at ways in which we can bring everything back together. Families become wretchedly fragmented over dealing with Alzheimer's, because of the difficulty of caring for the person who has the disease and because of family member's individual ways of interacting. Perhaps the most important fact for families to accept is that there is no perfect, no absolutely right, no unarguable way to deal with this disease. Every family's passage is inevitably going to be marked by disagreement and uncertainty.

Family members can often become very attached to their individual points of view, that is understandable, but underlying this attachment is often the secret conviction that doing things the "right" way will somehow change the course of Alzheimer's disease. This is what underlies so much of the anxiety and guilt among families affected by the disease.

"I just wish I knew the right thing to do," says Mitch of his father. "You know, if I could just make the right decisions then perhaps it'll stop what's happening."

Alzheimer's disease is an internal process. There is a level at that outer conditions affect it, but its main course is something within the victim. No one else can take it away, stop it, or even slow it down. Within each person, it has its own path and its own pace, responding to some internal timetable. Of course we should make life as easy and as comfortable as possible for the person who has this illness, but we need to accept that it is the other person's illness. We need to accept the present.

"I want my mother back," says Manny. "I don't want her to be this helpless little woman. My mother was strong and she looked after me and I want her back."

Manny's sense of loss and pain is understandable, but he cannot ever have that mother back. Either he accepts taking on the role of becoming father to his mother, or he continues to rage and sorrow about his loss. Because he does not cope, he fails to keep his appointments with social workers and others who could help him and enable his mother to have better care.

Many people with Alzheimer's consistently fail to get their needs met because their families are locked into trying to maintain who they used to be. One man tests his wife's memory every day to see if she can recall the names, addresses, and telephone numbers of their children. He is thrilled when she can but devastated when she fails. Actually, it is irrelevant whether she has a good memory on Tuesday—she definitely has Alzheimer's every day.

The person with Alzheimer's can have a great deal of happiness in the average day—but experiencing that happiness depends a great deal on the family. A lot can be done to make the present enjoyable for all concerned. Family members are often much sadder than the person who has the illness. The one good thing about Alzheimer's is that you can rely upon the here and now, although it can seem bizarre, especially if someone is under the impression that he is living in a time forty years ago. But bizarre need not be a problem. Happiness and sadness are the problems. Anxiety and grief are the problems.

If we love only the person who used to be, the person here and now gets no love from us. This is a very common situation in Alzheimer families: No one loves the person who is here now. That may seem a harsh way to describe the family's sadness and sense of loss, but it is nevertheless true.

When we say, "How can we help?" we have entered present time. We have stopped being trapped in the past. We have stopped fighting the disease and the person in the disease. We are ready and able to help. That is the start of reconciliation. We continue it by staying aware every day of what we are learning and how we are growing. This enables us to avoid being caught up in recrimination and struggle. We can learn to appreciate our own abilities and forgive our shortcomings. We are reconciled with who we are. Many people tormented by the Alzheimer situation are really being tormented by their own inner feelings of rage and guilt.

If we cannot accept our anger—the natural feelings that sometimes say, "I wish he were dead," or "How much longer is she going to live?"—then we become obsessed by guilt. Accepting our inner feelings allows us to come to oneness inside, instead of being torn apart by all kinds of opposing emotions. This is the powerful spiritual journey of caregiving. It forces us to be honest and it asks of us to accept and forgive, ourselves and others.

Acceptance and forgiveness are very important for the future of the family. Make no mistake—this is a disease that divides families forever, not a passing crisis soon over. A quick crisis can bring everyone close, but a long-term struggle allows each person to behave according to personal patterns of behavior. One will be a caregiver, someone else will be the organizer, someone else again will be the one who disappears whenever needed. If family members cannot learn to accept each other's levels of functioning, they may never speak to each other again.

It is hard for the one who does the caring to forgive those who do not, but it is less work in the long run. Holding grudges uses up valuable energy, and some people manage to make the decision not to use their energies in that way. Those who hold their anger close will be constantly torn up within; many stay permanently angry with Alzheimer's itself. Again, while understandable, this anger is a waste of time and energy. Alzheimer's is just a disease. It happens. Unfair things happen and we learn to cope or we don't. We can choose to do either.

The person interested in reconciliation will choose to cope, finding a way of making sense of the ordeal of Alzheimer's. We tend to be reluctant to accept another person's ordeal and in Alzheimer's, family members often project a sense of suffering that is not really there for the person who is ill. People suffer from imagined suffering much more than from suffering itself.

Following are some of the ways in that family caregivers have expressed their different views on making sense of Alzheimer's disease.

"In the end, my mother was just like a child. That was hard for us. She'd always been so competent and able to cope. Then there was this childlike clinging little girl. But, you know, she told me things then I never knew before. I learned that she had been frightened badly by her father. She used to come up to me and say, 'Don't let my daddy hurt me.' And I used to hold her and assure her she was safe. And sometimes I used to think, maybe this is what had to happen for her to finally find safety and love."

—MARGUERITE, age 49

"One thing that happened when we looked after our granddad was that my high school friends just loved him. He'd come out with some really weird, garbled ways of saying things and they loved that—they said he was like a mad poet. I thought that was kind of neat."

—ADAM, age 19

"My mother was always a real nag. She worried about everything. In the early stages of her illness, she was just awful, so anxious all the time. Later, she was so relaxed and happy. She'd sit out in the sunshine smiling in this blissful way. I could see she'd come to some place where she was more peaceful. Of course, she'd forgotten all the things she used to worry about. Even her hypertension got better."

—DICK, age 42

The issue of reconciliation becomes much more complicated when the initial relationship, prior to the illness, was a troubled one—when children, for example, are dealing with a sick parent who had many shortcomings as a parent. For some people, this is simply not an issue they can deal with.

> *"I can't look after my mother. I wouldn't put her into a home, but I'd never look after her myself. I just can't. She was never there for me as a child. She never behaved like my mother. She was always out working. She was a social worker and she spent all her time at work. I was looked after by hired girls. I can never get over that."*
>
> —MAUREEN, age 62

Maureen, fortunately, is wealthy. She pays an extraordinarily high wage to a caregiver who looks after her mother. She is doing the best she can and certainly she is obtaining the care her mother needs. Whether holding on to her anger and resentment will ultimately serve her is an issue she may come to deal with later.

Rosie took a different path, although some of her story is the same. "I could never stand my mother. She was always an angry, resentful woman who obviously didn't want to be a mother," she recalls. "I left home as soon as I could. I never went back until she was sick. Actually, I didn't know she was sick. I went to visit her for the first time in four or five years and I found her whole house in a squalid mess. It was really clear she couldn't manage."

Rosie got her mother to a doctor. After a long series of medical investigations, her mother was diagnosed with Alzheimer's disease.

"So then I had to think about what to do. It just seemed that there wasn't much choice at that moment. So I moved back in and started looking after her. Well, it was horrible. I still couldn't stand all the ways she was just like she used to be—and then there were a whole lot of new ways I couldn't stand either. She really drove me crazy. Well, it's kind of hard to explain but it just took up so much of my energy that I knew I had to give up, get out, and somehow change. And I changed. I just kind of let go of all those feelings I had about her. I hadn't got the strength to hold on any more to all that stuff."

From that time on, Rosie and her mother developed an entirely new kind of relationship.

"We became kind of like bad girls together. We'd go to the zoo sometimes or we'd sleep in late and not do our washing up till next day. The more I kind of relaxed, the more she changed. She even got quite a sense of humor. It was like she forgot what was bugging her all those years. And she forgot me. She could never get my name right. Once she said to me right out of the blue, 'Oh you should meet my daughter—she's a lovely girl,' and that was just great. I can only say I'm really glad I tried and it was really okay. My mother's dead now but I really feel good about what I did and how our life was in those last couple of years."

Rosie finally had to put her mother into care, and that was also a difficult choice.

"We were traveling at the time and she woke up one morning and there was nothing she could do. She couldn't dress, couldn't go to the bathroom, couldn't eat even. I felt real scared then. I knew it was over for us at that point. Well, I found a home for her, a small house where five old ladies lived. Her Social Security covered the cost and she fit right in. It was kind of a warm, down-homey place. I knew she'd be okay. I knew we were okay."

Another aspect of reconciliation that will concern family members is to make some reconciliation with the disease itself; otherwise they live in terror of it for the rest of their lives.

"Every time I forgot my keys, I thought, 'Oh God, that's it— it's happening to me now. I'm going to be just like my father.' I felt so scared and angry," relates one son.

These fears are extremely normal—and so too are those memory lapses. Losing keys, forgetting where you parked the car, searching for glasses—those are the usual memory lapses everyone experiences, including young people. But young people do not usually immediately think of Alzheimer's. Older people do.

A person could spend 20 years worrying about Alzheimer's and get run over by a truck at age 55 before the disease manifests. The most valuable thing each person can do is to fully develop his or her potential to live the fullest possible life and to work to overcome personal problems and issues. There is nothing else that we can really aim for that makes sense. As it happens, working on ourselves in this way, at emotional, spiritual, and intellectual levels, also makes us into more lovable people, and lovable people, if they need it, attract good caregivers.

This is not entirely a frivolous suggestion. In a 54-bed Alzheimer care unit in the San Francisco Bay Area, the residents who got the most love were the ones who were most lovable. They were easygoing, had a good sense of humor, were appreciative of others, and responsive to other people. These are characteristics that serve anyone well, in Alzheimer's or out.

One major reconciliation that family members need to undergo is one our whole society needs—the ability to cherish other people for their capacity to love and care, not for their intellect or power. Instead of being attached to our rational ways of valuing others, we need to develop our ability to love the other exactly as he or she is. This is not easy. Partners get disgusted with spouses who are demented. Children are frightened by parents who are no longer fully rational. We value people's independence and separateness. We need to learn to value what is there—the child that emerges.

"I learned to look at my husband a whole new way," Alice recalls. "I had to or go crazy. He couldn't run our life any more the way he used to. I had to do it. He got to goof off and do nothing or mess about, and I hated it. I wanted him back. I wanted the old age we had promised ourselves—our golden years of travel and fun."

Alice's husband became quite childlike. He wanted toys from the toy store. When his grandsons visited, he took their toys and refused to give them back. Finally, Alice gave in and bought him some toys of his own.

"And you know, one day I was watching him and, I'm really not a Christian, not a churchgoer, but I thought about that thing about being as little children and I said to myself, that's him. That's my Bill. And the funny thing is, once I could see him as the little boy he must have been, I felt as if that's who he was—a sweet, untouched little boy. It was like that part of him wasn't sick at all. Children don't get Alzheimer's, do they? I loved him in a new kind of way after that. He wasn't my husband any more but it didn't hurt quite as much because, after all, I still had him—that lovely boy."

In sacred writings, this emergence would be seen as the divine child who remains untouched by darkness or sickness.

For many caregivers this is one of the deep reconciliations that can come about.

"I looked after an old lady for a year," says one caregiver. "She wasn't a relative but I felt about her as if she were my grandmother. Even more, I could see the little girl in her—the way she wanted her daddy sometimes, the way she asked to go home to her daddy's house. I cherished her as if she were a little girl then and I didn't find it demeaning at all. She was a little child sometimes, just as we all are. Only it wasn't hidden away any more in her. You could see it."

Accepting the emergence of the child can be the most difficult thing for family members to do. Grown-ups are often disconcerted by childish or childlike behavior in adults. They are embarrassed at the betrayal. They want not to see it. And yet in a way it is one of the most whole parts of the person with Alzheimer's disease. With the emergence of the child can come a new sense of play, an emotional openness, a willingness to try new things and be real and authentic in all feelings, an ability to be free of judgment.

It is also an area that allows great healing, even within the disease process itself. Many people have suffered somewhat or greatly as children. Most people, throughout their lives, are working and reworking their primary relationships within themselves. This never stops until death itself. Particularly in old age comes a deep reworking of the primary issues of love, abandonment, wounding, and healing. This is why so many older people are preoccupied with their early lives. It is a normal part of maturation and reconciliation in life, of coming to peace.

It is exactly the same for the person with Alzheimer's, who is also deeply involved in those primary relationships, still trying to work them through and reach peace within. The main difference is that the person with Alzheimer's has often actually forgotten that those parent figures are dead, that this is some entirely different year from the one they are thinking about. That difference is not really as great as we might think. For most of us, the parent figures remain alive within us in the ways we play out our lives and our major relationships.

When the person with Alzheimer's reveals that he actually expects his mother to come home that night, the caregiver often focuses on the time error caused by dementia. We can help by concentrating instead on what is being said about the parent. We can focus on the feelings about the parent and the unresolved issues being talked about. We can help most of all by becoming an ideally loving parent figure so that the longing for love and safety and acceptance—common to all human beings—can actually be fulfilled in the here and now. By giving unconditional love now, we help heal the long-ago wounds of the past. By helping in that great healing, we give the same message to ourselves: No matter what the wound, we can all be healed.

We are learning about the deep nature of healing in the latter half of this century. We have all been brutally reminded that, after all, not all disease can necessarily be conquered, not all healing means recovery or even survival. We are being forced to ask ourselves how we may be healed. We have been learning that not all healing means not dying. Sometimes it means finding peace before we die.

Alzheimer's Communication— Following Clues

....

There is a science and an art in every human communication, and both are needed when dealing with people who have Alzheimer's disease. Basic communication is heavily impaired in this disease, presumably because physical damage to the brain impedes normal message-passing in the brain system. It becomes hard for people to formulate and express complex thoughts, and rational thinking is obstructed. This shows in many ways: the person mishears or misinterprets what is said; the meaning of words may be disconnected from their sound; even if the person hears accurately, it may be impossible for the person to construct a logical sentence for reply; even if the capacity to think cognitively is present, the speech center of the brain may not obey the person's wishes and the wrong words may emerge, as happens to stroke victims. We may never know which of the communication processes is actually dysfunctional, because the person may be unable to reply intelligibly or may suffer from "word salad," speaking a stream of apparent nonsense.

These obstacles can lead to many roadblocks in normal communication. In fact, the person with Alzheimer's is like someone dealing with a damaged computer—parts of the program are missing, and without the support and structure supplied by these missing bits of programming, the person is left trying to make sense of a world that seems crazy. The single most important thing to remember about all this is that the person with Alzheimer's disease is not crazy. Every communication has a purpose, and our task as caregivers is to find out what that is.

Nothing is meaningless—no word, no action. Even what sounds like nonsense, even the continuous repetition of the same sentence or question, is intended to express a feeling, to show a need, to give information, or to get a response. As caregivers, we need to remind ourselves constantly that Alzheimer-afflicted people are trying to understand everyday life, just as we are. We all want to make sense of things. That is the basis of most therapy—to make sense of our story. If strange or distressing events happen to us in daily life, we ask ourselves what is going on. If people behave in puzzling ways, we ask what they mean by them. People with Alzheimer's are doing the same thing.

The difference is that an essential part of their information system has been disabled. It is like being a stranger in a strange land, not understanding the customs nor speaking the language very well. Having Alzheimer's is like becoming that stranger without having consciously or knowingly gone into unknown territory. Instead, everything that is familar and loved about life becomes strange, unknown, and therefore often frightening. Even the people we love become strangers, since we may not be able to name them correctly or place them in context.

Staying aware of this as the central issue of Alzheimer's communication helps remind us to always ask ourselves: "What is the need being expressed by this behavior?" When language and function betray the sick, leaving them without the ability to say what they mean, the only thing left is action. Acting out becomes a symbolic portrayal of their truth. For example, people who constantly wander away from home may be acting out the fear they are trying to flee or the displacement they express by going off to find "home" again.

People with this disease are constantly acting out their needs and their feelings within a fractured brain structure. This means as caregivers we often witness apparently bizarre behavior or are confronted with peculiar demands. Stressed-out caregivers often fall into blaming the person at this point, simply because the complexities of communication are too overwhelming, added to everything else that has to be taken care of. As one wife said, "You know, there are days when I really don't give a damn what he needs. I just think, he's okay because he's got me, but who cares about my needs?"

That caregiver's reactions are very understandable. Why indeed should we bother so much about what someone with Alzheimer's really means? The main reason is that the sick person will inevitably continue to react negatively if his or her needs are not met and thus will increase caregiver load. This is not, by the way, deliberate on their part. It is instinctual reaction, just like the sunflower following the sun.

Therefore, our task is to decode the communication and to meet the need being expressed. Caregivers could use this mantra: No Alzheimer communication is meaningless. This applies whether the communication takes the form of words or actions. Most caregivers report the highest amount of stress arises when the person they are looking after is doing or saying things that do not make sense. In many workshops, caregivers find resolution once they begin to comprehend what certain speech and behavior actually signify.

Even in care facilities—and sometimes especially in care facilities—the real expressed needs of the person with Alzheimer's are virtually ignored. Being unlistened to is one of the major factors in creating what are usually described as problem behaviors. It is often the main impetus in outbreaks of violence when they do occur. In years of dealing with Alzheimer sufferers in private homes, home care residences, and skilled nursing facilities, I have never come across a problem behavior that did not arise from unmet needs or poor handling by caregivers. This aspect of Alzheimer care is neglected, undoubtedly because no one likes to criticize a caregiver who is already overburdened. However, it is time to talk about this, since ignoring this central issue actually leads to most of the major difficulties in caring for a person with Alzheimer's. The sufferer feels alone, and this results in what others define as difficult behaviors, which lead to most of the placements into full-time care.

It would be useful to drop the term difficult behaviors, since that phrase makes them the fault of the person who is sick, instead of reminding us that there may be better ways for us to listen, observe, and respond. Searching for the meaning of the behavior pays off, sometimes dramatically, and helps families to relate better. One woman reports, "My mother drove me crazy by always asking where the children were. I'd tell her, then she'd ask again. Eventually I realized this was her only way of being able to start a conversation. It really just meant she wanted to talk."

Once this woman was able to see her mother's annoyingly repeated question as a sort of verbal "ahem," it no longer bothered her. Most Alzheimer sufferers feel alone trying to communicate what they want and feel. Some family members may find it hard to give time to solving behavior problems and, in many other cases, dealing with the real issues of communication may involve more honesty and risk than family members are willing to face. This is understandable, but if they do not make the effort, they will certainly become overwhelmed by caregiving.

It is common for people with Alzheimer's to drop the use of nouns altogether, including personal names. Often a sentence comes out sounding very gnomic indeed because of the lack of nouns. For example, one woman said after a walk, "The little ones are very tired." At first, her caregiver thought she meant she was tired, but then the woman rubbed her foot painfully and repeated, "These little ones are tired now." When the caregiver removed the woman's shoes, she found that her toes had been skinned by ill-fitting shoes. The "little ones" were her toes, which were sore.

These constant roadblocks to communication are wearisome to both parties, and it is caregiver weariness that leads to most Alzheimer placements into professional care. It is not because people need such care—in fact, skilled nursing care is often extremely inappropriate for dementia patients. People are put into care because their caregivers are worn out. They are put into care because families cannot deal with the real issues of their illness, typically undealt-with anger, grief, secrecy about the illness, unaccepted role changes, control problems, and inability to nurture.

This chapter takes the widest possible interpretation of communication, acknowledging what linguists and social researchers tell us: that only 30 percent of human communication is verbal, and the rest is symbolically expressed through body language, actions, and behaviors. Begin your understanding by listening to what the person says and responding or interacting kindly.

When you speak with a person who is deeply impaired by Alzheimer's, speak in sentences that are clear and simple, in a voice that is soft and kind, in a manner that is unhurried and relaxed. Sharp voices agitate; hurry causes nervousness and dysfunction; complexity causes intellectual overload, which will bring about a distress response that could be rage, tears, anxiety, or extreme slowness and inability to do tasks. Speak on the same level as the person, both literally so you can be face to face, and figuratively so that you express ideas in a way that can be easily absorbed.

No one likes to be patronized, and people with Alzheimer's resent it as much as anyone else. As caregivers we always need to remind ourselves that, just because people have Alzheimer's disease, it does not mean they are either insensitive or stupid. They are functionally impaired, not stupid, and they are often highly aware of their own and other people's feelings. They may sometimes say things that we would consider inappropriate and hurtful—"Oh, you're very fat, aren't you?"—but this is due to unlearning the societal inhibitors they were taught when young.

Be sure to approach the person from the front so you can be seen. Surprises are not welcome in the world of dementia. Speak clearly, give plenty of time for the other person to respond, and avoid memory questions. To be sure you have the person's attention, gently place your hand on his or her arm, hand, or shoulder and be sure you have eye contact. Persons with Alzheimer's often spend periods of time in altered consciousness and they need to be gently brought back into the here and now.

It is astonishing how many caregivers think it appropriate to ask a person with severe memory problems all kinds of questions involving memory. Here is, unfortunately, a typical family dialogue:

"Hi, Ma, how are you? Do you know who I am? No, not Vonnie, that was your brother. Why would you think I was your brother, Ma? Do you know the names of your other children? Huh? Well, what did you do today, Ma? What did you have for breakfast? Look, do you know who this is? Huh, Ma?"

If this man could accept his mother's Alzheimer's disease, the greeting might be much less distressing for all concerned if it went as follows: "Hi, Ma, it's me, your son Ron. Good to see you. Boy, you look pretty nice today. Let's see, it's about five now. They'll be bringing your dinner at six, so that gives me enough time to show you some photos we took last week."

This communication works better because it does not constantly put Ron's mother to the test. It also considerately supplies linkage and potentially missing information and it keeps emphasis on the here and now. The photographs will give Ron a chance to identify other important family members and to remind his mother that they exist and they love her. The past is a murky country for the Alzheimer's sufferer and the future has often become unimaginable, but the present is always with us. Therefore, we can always rely on the present to be a part of our communication that can be fully shared.

Just as when we meet a stranger at a social gathering, we need to introduce ourselves afresh each time we meet a person with Alzheimer's disease. Here is another common example of a distressful communication: "You remember me, don't you? Can you tell me what my name is? Do you remember what we did last week? We really enjoyed ourselves. Don't tell me you've forgotten already."

This would be much less distressing rephrased as, "Hello, Irene, I'm Sally. I met you last week at the center and we had a lot of fun dancing together. My goodness, you're a really good dancer, aren't you?"

Relatives too should learn this social skill of introducing themselves. This will help to remove some of their distress when their husband or father or mother cannot get their name right. It is not personal, not an attack on their individuality. It is merely due to the disease's attack on the brain of the sufferer. Memory capacity varies from day to day, literally, and there will be better days and worse ones.

Conversational chit-chat can remain as a good social skill even among the deeply afflicted. This can lead distant family members to assume that the person is in better shape than he or she really is. A typical family miscommunication along this line might be as follows:

MARY

Mom, this is April on the telephone.

MOM

April?

79

MARY

Yes, your daughter April. She's my younger sister.

MOM

Well, who are you?

MARY

I'm your oldest daughter. Now, come on, April's here on the telephone.

[Mom heads into the kitchen because she has no idea what the word telephone represents anymore. Mary retrieves Mom and leads her to the telephone. Mom puts the wrong end of the receiver to her ear and Mary puts it the right way up.]

MARY

Say, hi April.

MOM

Hi, April.

APRIL

Oh Mom, it's so good to hear your voice. You sound great. How are you doing?

MOM

I'm doing fine.

APRIL

So did you go to Henry's for Thanksgiving?

MOM

Yes. [Actually she did not.]

APRIL

That's great. Did you enjoy yourself?

MOM

Yes.

APRIL

Well, Bill and I are fine and...

Two minutes after this conversation ends, Mom has forgotten entirely that there was a call, and April is telling Bill that Mom sounds fine and she cannot possibly be doing as badly as Mary always says she is.

A number of other major problems in communication concern memory issues. We do not really understand how deeply we are tied into our memory structure until we live with someone who is not. Then we see that the loss of reliable memory function fractures the whole of life. Caregivers who are confronted by this often find themselves frustrated, sometimes hurt, and often caught up in uncomfortable exchanges that result in bad communication. These appear constantly in the questions raised by caregivers in Alzheimer workshops: "My dad has no idea what year this is. I think he thinks it's about 1925 and he calls me by his brother's name. What should I do?"

The major loss in memory dysfunction is knowing what year this is. Memory is like a ship, anchored to the current year, and when it loses that anchor entirely we never know from one moment to the next what year that person's memory has drifted into. To the person with Alzheimer's, memories feel as real as experience of the here and now.

Rather than designating this as a delusion, it is more useful to consider it as a loss of reference system. When confronted by a parent whose memory ship may have floated back to age 16 in Texas, acceptance can be very calming. If the son explains that this is 1993 and he is not his father's younger brother, this information may not be acceptable or understandable. It may seem as if a time machine has suddenly landed from the future. Experimentation is the answer. If his father can accept gentle reorienting to the here and now, that is good. If he does not accept it or seems uninterested, then the son needs to accept his father's drift of memory.

81

One area of communication that puzzles and often hurts family members is their misidentification. A son is thought to be a brother or father; a daughter is called sister or mother; wives are thought to be mother; husbands are called daddy. These misidentified relatives feel rejected and hurt. However, if they could put themselves into that frustrating Alzheimer brain, they might see that, first, the ability to label a person correctly has been destroyed. Second, if the memory ship has drifted to the past, to premarriage days, then it makes sense that they cannot be spouse or child in that particular memory picture. Third, when they are named as the parent, the person is really saying, "I love you and I need your love and care and protection as a child needs his parent." When they are named as a sibling, the person is saying, "I know you are very near and related to me."

Confrontation as communication leads to hostility and misunderstanding and never achieves what the caregiver wants to achieve, which is usually either to stop the person from doing something, or alternatively, to make that person do some desired action. Usually when confrontation occurs, it comes out of the caregiver's anxiety, hurry, or hostility, and these are probably additional reasons why it fails. Persons with Alzheimer's are very sensitive and they pick up even underlying unstated angers and fears.

Instead of confronting, think of how you would get a small child to cooperate. You would be kind, persuasive, and patient, ideally. Use these same skills and make sure you always allow enough time. Instead of saying, "No, you can't do that," use diversion, bribery, and food. Say, "I really need you to help me over here right now," and lead the person away from danger or trouble.

If you have confronted the person, with unwanted results, ask yourself if you were actually feeling hostile at the moment you did it. Probably you were. In our hurry and need, we sometimes forget to treat people we look after with dignity and respect. We want to demand instant obedience and get the situation over and done with.

Another major communication problem in families is the big question of whether to tell The Awful Truth. This is often raised in workshops and support groups. A husband asks,

"Should I tell my wife she has Alzheimer's disease?" A wife asks, "When is the right time to say something to him about his illness? I don't want to hurt him."

Family members mean well when they say nothing. They fear that they will hurt, frighten, or depress the person concerned, and so no one ever mentions the dreaded word Alzheimer's. This kind of thinking has been pretty much exploded now in other medical fields. Numerous studies have shown that people not only want to know what is wrong with them, they are actually relieved to hear the truth even when the news is bad. This is as true in Alzheimer's as it is in cancer, Huntington's chorea, and other serious illnesses. People are so stressed by knowing that something is wrong, even though no one talks about it, that the truth is a great relief and a great release.

There is absolutely no chance that a person who has been slowly developing Alzheimer's over the years has not noticed that something is terribly wrong. Usually, in the past, before Alzheimer awareness had developed, people thought they were either going crazy or becoming unaccountably stupid. However they described it, they knew without a doubt that something was profoundly wrong with them. If we never speak of the illness to them, we condemn them to live in a lonely place of silence. If we want to be good caregivers, we will release them from being so alone. Caregivers who refuse to tell the truth need to look deeply into their own motivation, beyond the expressed wish to spare someone else pain, into the problem of their own pain.

Nowadays, most people working in the Alzheimer's field meet people who have already accurately suspected that this is what is wrong with them. Although it is frightening, they are relieved to be able to speak about what is happening, and they can then try to develop ways of dealing with some aspects of the disease. The caregiver who tells the truth is not taking away hope. In fact, those who wish to deny their illness will manage to do so in the face of all family insistence. It is impossible to take away denial from those who really wish to hide behind it.

As people become more deeply impaired by Alzheimer's, they find it harder to complete the tasks of daily living. They often need constant verbal cueing to do things like get dressed or take a shower. The main thing to remember about any such cueing is that it must be done one step at a time. Memory failure means the person cannot keep a number of actions in mind. Give one instruction at a time and point to the objects you name: "Here, Annie, why don't you put on this sock? That's it. That's great. Now this one. Good. Now here's your sneaker. And here's the other one."

Constant conversational accompaniment can be very soothing. Never give orders, always make suggestions. Never insist. Always back off if there is a problem and return to it in a few moments. Never try to hurry anyone through step-by-step procedures. Hurry causes dysfunction. If the person resists a procedure, ask yourself if this is necessary and drop it if it is not. If it is essential, try bribery. A dish of ice cream, a cookie, or a piece of cake can be a soothing communication device. Be specific—for example, "Here's some great strawberry ice cream," not "What kind of ice cream would you like?" Never offer more than two choices.

Preferably the conversation should be referring to an actual object in the room. The danger of referring to absent objects is that you have no way of knowing for sure that the words you use are being understood by the person you are speaking to. A sample of this confusion:

"Hilda, we have some really nice lentil soup today. Would you like some?" offers the caregiver, but without showing Hilda the soup.

"Oh yes," says Hilda enthusiastically.

Given a generous serving of soup, Hilda eats with obvious and increasing reluctance and distaste.

"Hilda, I notice you aren't eating the soup. Is there something wrong?"

"Oh yes, it's terrible, just terrible!"

Since the soup was actually delicious, the caregiver realized that lentil soup was simply something that Hilda did not enjoy eating. Checking with a family member confirmed that Hilda had always hated lentil soup.

A more constructive exchange would be the following:

"Here's some nice tomato soup, Hilda. Do you think you'd like a bowl?" asks the caregiver, showing Hilda the pan of soup. Hilda looks in, recognizes the contents as something she likes, and agrees she would like this. And she does.

Most impaired people cannot choose appropriate clothing for the day, yet it is pleasant to involve them in the process of picking what they will wear. Show, for example, two sweaters and ask, "Would you like this one or that one today?" If you do not want to deal with choices, then offer items with a strong suggestion that manipulates toward your choice.

"This sweater always looks so pretty on you, Hilda. Would you like to wear it today?" will usually elicit the answer "yes."

In the same way, when your charge asks you difficult questions that lead to problems, you will soon learn how to evade, concur, or be conversationally noncommittal. This may cause dilemmas for you at first. Most of us want honesty in our communication with others. We do not feel good about lying, rightly so. However, in dementia, we are often presented with situations that specifically bring up issues in which blatant literal honesty causes great pain and confusion. For example, a weeping 88-year-old woman says, "Why hasn't my mother been to see me? I haven't seen her for a long time." Even if told the truth that her mother is dead, she will usually reject the information because she is not living in the present reality, and you cannot maker her do so.

If you believe that reality orientation is the one honest way to go, you may tell this human being who desperately needs mothering that her mother is dead. This is neither necessary, relevent, nor kind, and it tends to bring about catastrophic reactions of grief, rage, or heated denial. It is profoundly necessary for caregivers of people with dementia to understand that we must respect their reality; it is not their duty to come into our reality. It is only the inexperienced, rigid, or unkind caregiver who sticks to ramming unpleasant so called "real" facts down the throats of lonely, frightened old people.

No one can forcibly change the reality of a person with Alzheimer's. Often, the demented person knows emotionally exactly what is needed and will not be distracted from that need. The displaced one wants to go home, even if he is sitting in his own home. The one who feels useless and unwanted wants to cook dinner or clean up the house that is no longer hers and may not even exist any more. The frightened lonely one wants mother. Just as small children only want what they want, with a deep emotional intensity, so too do those with Alzheimer's. Reality orientation is meaningless because they are expressing their feelings, not concerns about facts.

A perceptive and kindly caregiver soon begins to learn that dealing with the emotional needs presented by the person is a much more useful way to go. To the woman who wants to know where her mother is, the caregiver might say, "I'm not sure right now [this will almost certainly be true], but maybe you'd like to have some coffee with me and we can sit and read together."

To the woman who says she is expected at home, the caregiver might say sympathetically, "Are you feeling lonely right now?" or "I guess you're really missing your family right now. I'm sorry," then offer some attractive distraction.

The basic rule in communicating with people presenting their own demented reality is, first, acknowledge their feelings and, second, do something about their needs, either in offering emotional support and security or by distracting them into something that helps them let go of the feeling for a while.

What about the person who is offering an entirely different reality in the form of an interesting fantasy life? This is not uncommon though it is more usual for people to go back in time, either to traumas that tormented them or, more commonly, to happy times and pleasant events. In the case of people who basically are simply reviewing their lives and coming to resolution, caregivers need only offer empathy and support.

One woman in a day-care program repeatedly told the story of her first day at school when she wet her pants and was humiliated by the teacher in front of everyone. Some caregivers regularly laughed at this, reinforcing her feelings of humiliation. Others belittled the story—"Oh you worry too much, Elsie"—thus denying her feelings. It does not take great perception to understand several things about Elsie's story. The first important point, which none of the caregivers picked up, is that the day-care experience was in itself triggering the memory—new surroundings, new faces, insecurity, fear of humiliation, probably actual fear of not getting to the bathroom in time. Second, because the caregivers were failing to respond appropriately to her need, Elsie was condemned to repetition of her story. The more useful response might have been an acknowledgment of her feelings, followed by reassurance:—"Oh Elsie, what a terrible thing to happen to you on your first day at school. That teacher was wrong to treat you that way. She should have helped you. It's quite different here. We're your friends here and I'll show you exactly where the bathroom is. You needn't worry about that."

Caregivers need to be ready to respond appropriately however often the story is told. It is not memory loss that causes Elsie to repeat her story, except in a superficial sense. It is the continuing pain and fear she feels. Take care of her needs at the feeling level and she will no longer need to repeat her story. It will be exorcised, leaving her free to return to more pleasant memories. Many people stick with their happy memories. One old lady who lived in a nursing home gave birth to babies every night. She was overcome with joy and triumph, and her happiness was so clear to the staff that eventually everyone joined in and supported her. Staff would look in on her and say, "How's that baby coming, Grace?"

This brings us to the dilemma of re-created reality. It is one thing to agree to support people's feelings about real events in the past and even to accept that they are reexperiencing those events in an emotionally real but not factual sense in the present. However, a number of people with Alzheimer's create an entirely new past and present. Again, we could label this with psychiatric jargon as delusion and hallucination, but that does not get us anywhere, except to give us a vocabulary. A vocabulary does not, however, give us the tools to deal with the person. For that we need not words but our own feelings of empathy.

People besieged by Alzheimer's go through great pain, fear, and loss at various stages. Therefore, when we see them creating brand-new interesting and rewarding fantasy lives for themselves, we should recognize this as a coping device, a way of making the unbearable bearable—even a way of telling the self an interesting story, making a new life when the old one was not fulfilling many needs. We all need to dream. Having Alzheimer's does not remove this need, although it may remove the cognitive ability to divide dream from actuality.

There are probably more people in convalescent hospitals and care homes with these new realities than people at home. That is because emotional and spiritual life in such places is much more bleak for those forced to live in them. They are taken from a real life of their own, however impaired, and given instead a restrictive regime devised by someone else and modeled on a sterile medical mode of containment. Often people have nothing or little to do in such places, so they create their own amusement. One 84-year-old woman, Rosie, was married once, widowed and childless. In an Alzheimer's unit she developed a rich new life in which she had been married seven times and had 21 children and was currently pregnant. Another woman, Maria, was 95, a devout Roman Catholic with a large Mexican family who seldom came to see her. Soon after being moved into a nursing home, she began carrying around a doll that she said was the Baby Jesus. Richard, a man who had always done many home repairs, walked around the Alzheimer's unit where he lived, carrying out invisible tasks of repair. He even took an invisible dog for walks sometimes. His actions were so authentic that one nurse swore she could almost see the dog.

Some professionals feel that people with dementia should have their invented realities adjusted to factual life, forcibly if necessary. However, this can never be done successfully. It seems far more humane and considerate simply to accept that this is their chosen reality. Most professionals who work with the demented adjust to accepting their reality, if only because the patients hold on to it so fiercely that any attempt to take it away only causes tears and tantrums. In rare instances, re-created realities cause problems, as in the case of the man who felt that neighbors were about to break into his house, whereupon he became very violent. However, his fears arose out of the terror and loneliness of his disease, which his wife refused to discuss with him.

If we are good parents, we do not tell young children they are liars when they come to us with stories of talking dogs and friendly giants and adventures flying on butterfly backs. We understand that they have imagination and a story they want to tell. We owe at least as much understanding to those who are working through their dementia in ways that bring them pleasure or consolation.

People with dementia have two needs of us in our communication with them. They need us to respect the adult in them as well as to honor the child. Instead of feeling, as many family members do, that it is demeaning to see an adult operating in some aspects at a child level, perhaps instead we can come to understand that the child within does not get Alzheimer's. Therefore, if we can work with the child that emerges as the disease progresses, we can ease the pain and loneliness of this difficult journey. If we can acknowledge the physics professor's new ability to paint as freely and inventively as a child, instead of bemoaning the fact that his great computing mind is damaged beyond repair, we can do more for him in the average day than everyone who mourns the lost professor.

We will get the cues in the language those with Alzheimer's use to us. If the impaired adult wants mother, father, brother, we know he feels lonely and insecure. If he asks to go home or back to the Texas he left as a youth, we know he feels lost and displaced. If we can find ways to offer the accepting and unchanging love of the ideal mother, father, brother, if we can create a world that welcomes him and helps him feel at home, that person will be much happier and much more resolved.

Language is likely to fail gradually as the disease progresses. The person uses names less often, if ever—something that may happen even in the early phases. Nouns used abstractly may not be connected to their meaning any more. The person may be unable to find the words needed.

"Could you buy me one of those—you know—small and I had two in my refrigerator but now there's only one," turns out to be a request for lamb chops—which, by the way, the caregiver understood.

Language connections may be lost, either because of memory failure—the inability to hold a sentence in mind so it can be completed—or because of brain dysfunction, so that rational thoughts literally cannot go through the right neuropathways. Sentences may stay uncompleted or become very convoluted as the person follows around determinedly but cannot get quite the right words and phrases.

"I think that something soon will happen that is terrible if something soon is not done," was Hilda's way of saying "I urgently need to get to the bathroom."

As caregivers, therefore, we will make intuitive jumps, guesses, and mistakes as we try to understand. If someone really cannot tell us what is wanted, we can try to be empathetic. It is important to let that person know we really want to understand the frustration. If we cannot understand, finally, we can say, "I'm really sorry I don't understand what you need. I'll try harder."

Gradually, the impaired person may say less and less and seem to be further and further away. This awayness, which is certainly some kind of being in an altered state, often goes on for longer and longer, especially toward the end stages of the disease. None of us knows where people go to in these states, but we do know from brain studies that people with Alzheimer's dream much more than most people and also show a great deal of brain wave activity. The insensitive person may simply say, as one man did of his mother, "There's no one home anymore. I mean, she's just dead really. She's a living corpse."

However, most caregivers who develop a good understanding of the Alzheimer process do not agree with this estimation. Instead, they tend to say, as one nurse did, "I don't where she goes but I know for sure she goes somewhere. I sit next to her and I can see that she's far away somewhere doing something. Then she comes back and she's there again."

This sense of interior preoccupation is often found in those in the later stages of Alzheimer's. They give the impression, not of being the living dead, but of being the absorbed absentee away doing other things. It never seems to be a distressed state, always one of quiet absorption. Some people in such states have even been taken to hospital, as one Jungian therapist with severe Alzheimer's was, only to be sent home diagnosed as being in an altered state.

If someone seems to be in this state, usually shown by being very quietly deep in thought and unaware of the here and now, it is good to sit quietly and await the person's return. It is better not to interrupt or break into this state of reverie, since that can be experienced as disruptive or frightening. Their awayness should be respected. You can even explore it by asking the person where he or she has been. The answers can be interesting, though not necessarily very comprehensible.

Use physical contact as your constant message that everything is all right and that you love the person. It is rare for people to find such touch unwelcome, but if they indicate this, respect it.

For most people, touch is a message that gets through when words do not. Lay your hand on the person's arm when you talk, gently rub her back, massage his shoulders, give a hand massage. Any such physical movement should be slow, firm, and leisurely. Quick pats and tugs are very disturbing and unpleasant. If a hug is appropriate and welcome, a side-by-side hug is less threatening than a full frontal body hug, which can be very invasive. Do not use hugging as a way of patronizing people; they will detect your insincerity.

Some of your communication may concern the setting of limits. It is important to be able to set limits, even if the person cannot remember them. It is appropriate to say to someone who is being verbally abusive, "I'm sorry you feel like that but I don't care to be spoken to this way." Such words do not necessarily stop the person with Alzheimer's, but they will make you feel less powerless.

Setting limits is not the same as trying to retrain someone. Forget about that entirely. Trying to retrain someone with Alzheimer's is one of the things that family members find it hard to let go of.

A husband reports, "I tell her not to go into the kitchen but she's always sneaking in there, and I can't trust her anymore."

The answer is not to forbid the wife the kitchen in which she has worked for 35 years. It is to make the kitchen Alzheimer-proof.

A wife says, "My biggest problem right now is trying to get my husband to stop answering the phone when I'm out. I keep telling him."

Yes, but having Alzheimer's means he keeps forgetting. Her solution must be not to change him but to turn off the telephone ringer and get a quiet answering machine.

The basis of all our communication in Alzheimer's disease should be empathetic understanding, receptivity, intuition and loving kindness. If we use them all constantly, we will understand much, reach out more, and become the true companions that are so needed and yearned for by those who journey through this darkness.

The key to the puzzle usually lies in listening with the heart.

Getting Through the Day— Daily Problem-Solving

....

"When we function from this place of spacious awareness rather than our analytic mind, we are often surprised to find solutions to problems without our having 'figured them out.'"
—RAM DASS & PAUL GORMAN, *How Can I Help?*

Sometimes caregivers feel as if the whole of caring for some-one with Alzheimer's is one problem after another. It is true that the caregiver's main task is the constant search for solutions. This chapter is intended to help you look for ways of coping with problems. The solutions may be obvious or they may require some innovative thinking or adjustment on your part. Not all problems necessarily have a solution that puts a stop to them. Sometimes the answer will be to try to change yourself.

There is only one major thing to remember: All Alzheimer behaviors have meaning. Your task as a caregiver is to try to find that meaning and meet the need expressed by it. This can be difficult. After all, this disease is a dementia, but the sufferer is trying to make sense of an increasingly bewildering world; the resulting behaviors are intended to communicate.

Brain function impairment gives rise to certain patterns of behavior, such as, repeating questions or constantly pacing about, but the exact nature of the behavior usually represents a need the person is trying to have met. Let us look at a typical irritating behavior. Many people with Alzheimer's ask repetitive questions. "What time is it?" or "Can I go home now?" or "Where are my mother and father?" The questions are repeated over and over because the person can remember neither asking previously nor receiving the answer. However, as you will see in the section below headed "Repetitive Questions," there is often a deeper issue involved, which you must uncover before you can stop those irritating questions. When you meet the real needs of the person with Alzheimer's, you will find resolution and the possibility of living in emotional peace with each other.

This may sound as if you, the caregiver, have to make all the compromises. To a great extent, that is true. Since the person with Alzheimer's cannot work from a fully functioning brain, the caregiver does indeed have to find solutions. If that seems unfair, remember that it is also very hard work to be the one who has Alzheimer's. It is frightening, lonely, and frustrating for the sufferer. Out of that come most of the angers, tears, and difficult behaviors that you have to deal with. As a caregiver, you will find many solutions once you understand a behavior.

Be sure you are honest about who has the problem. Many problem behaviors are only a problem to the caregiver. They do not cause any embarrassment, inconvenience, or risk to the person with Alzheimer's. Being clear about this will help you find solutions that meet your needs without causing you to come into conflict with the Alzheimer's sufferer. For example, if the problem is someone undressing inappropriately indoors, you could close the curtains rather than fight about getting dressed again. This may not be the answer you wanted, but it may be the best workable solution.

The fact that the behavior is a problem for you and not for the person with Alzheimer's does not make it not worth solving. As the caregiver, you must try to make life as pleasant for yourself as you can. It is hard enough looking after someone with Alzheimer's as it is. You do not have to accept the unacceptable. You just have to be clear about the reality of the situation and the nature of the problem.

The rest of this chapter is arranged alphabetically by problem. If you cannot find what you are looking for, check the index for further information.

DAILY PROBLEM-SOLVING

ABUSE

The old woman was sitting on a hospital gurney, waiting to be seen by the duty doctor. Her face was swollen and she had two black eyes. An X-ray technician stopped beside her.

"Oh my, what happened to you? Did you fall over?"

The old woman smiled. "Oh no," she said cheerfully.

"But your eyes are black and blue!" exclaimed the technician.

"Oh well," said the old woman vaguely, "I suppose someone must have painted them."

That is an excellent example of why people with Alzheimer's are in special need of protection from abuse. They may have no memory of abuse. They cannot communicate clearly, and not everyone has the patience to decode what they say.

Abuse of the elderly is as unadmitted now as abuse of children used to be. Alzheimer's Association statistics say that up to four percent of the elderly are being abused. Given that figures say four million Americans have Alzheimer's disease, that means some 160,000 elders with Alzheimer's are being abused.

Unfortunately, abuse and Alzheimer's disease do go together. It is a very stressful disease for caregivers to cope with. This can bring out the kinds of feelings that lead to abuse. Abuse can occur in a number of ways—physical, emotional, sexual, financial, as well as abuse through neglect and illegal restraint.

The person with Alzheimer's is particularly helpless against abuse, and caregivers have a moral as well as a legal duty to protect anyone who is helpless to assert personal rights. If you suspect that family abuse of any kind is going on, you must contact your local elder services agency. Medical and social work professionals are also required to report abuse so that intervention can help everyone concerned. Nurses and doctors are required to make abuse reports when marks of violence are found on their patients.

This is a new field of awareness, so there are few figures available. However, almost every Area Agency on Aging in the country now has an elder abuse hotline listed in its resources, and doctors and emergency room personnel are being trained to look for signs of abuse. They are the same signs in elders in children—bruises, falls, broken bones, none of which can be clearly accounted for. Even the suspicion of abuse can now lead to reports being made to senior and disabled services agencies for further investigation. It is an issue just beginning to surface.

One of the more dramatic stories to emerge that basically qualifies as abuse was the story of Oregonian Sue Gifford, charged with abandoning her elderly father who had Alzheimer's disease. She took him out of state and abandoned him in his wheelchair at a racetrack on the other side of the country, with a note falsifying his name. He was recognized in the newspapers by the staff of the care home where he had been residing. Although more dramatic than most, it was a story that typified the many issues usually concerned in abuse. The daughter had been long estranged from her father and had personal and emotional problems that led to the action of abandonment. She claimed that her alcoholic father had sexually and physically abused her when she was young. The fact that she was placed on probation indicates that the court was made aware of the complexity of issues involved.

Such problems seldom come about because an abuser is just plain cruel. It is usually a combination of factors that causes people to injure those who need their help and protection. Overwhelming situations combined with personal inadequacies are the usual components. Most medical personnel and social workers can well understand the pressures that can lead to abuse. Their concern is to help the family cope. If you know that you are being abusive, or in danger of becoming so, get help immediately from your local senior services agency.

It is natural to feel angry at someone you are always looking after, but it is entirely wrong to hit, push, or physically punish that person. It is normal to feel like yelling sometimes, but you have to find ways to express those impulses without being abusive to the person in your charge. For example, you could go for a ride in your car, wind up the windows and yell as you drive. You might feel strange about that, but better out than in when it comes to emotional pressure.

Once it starts, abuse escalates, so get help before it starts. Get counseling, ask for help from any local office concerned with care for the elderly, go to support groups, and learn to laugh instead of getting mad.

Of course, not all abuse is physical or emotional. In Alzheimer's it is not unusual for financial abuse to occur, with a family or sometimes even an outside caregiver taking financial advantage of the incompetent person. This must also be reported by anyone who suspects it, and action can be taken by the justice system and by the social services system to safeguard the assets of an incompetent person.

Rarely can a demented person accurately identify being abused. However, it is fairly common for someone with Alzheimer's to claim that he or she is being abused when it is not true. People may accuse others of stealing from them, of not feeding them, even of hitting or beating them when it is entirely untrue. This obviously complicates the issues. Concerned people should keep an eye open for physical evidence that may suggest abuse, while also staying aware of the fact that any of these can result from legitimate accidents.

Sam and his wife Marge took care of Sam's mother, who had Alzheimer's. They took her for an Alzheimer's workup and found themselves being reported to the local senior services agency for abuse when bruise marks were found on her arm. They had never abused her. She was prone to easy bruising, as many older people are, and had probably acquired the marks when being helped up from a low armchair. The accusations shattered the couple, and soon after they placed Sam's mother in a care home. This sad story highlights the complexity of the abuse issue—one where we cannot exaggerate the dangers enough and yet must always be aware of witch-hunts.

AGITATION

Many people with Alzheimer's have periods of agitation when they become anxious, worried, obsessive, fearful, or angry to a considerable degree. It is common for this to occur in the late afternoon, typically between 3 P.M. and 7 P.M. This phenomenon is not peculiar to Alzheimer's disease. It is associated with many dementias and can also happen to older people who otherwise seem to be in good health. These late-afternoon periods of emotional agitation are often referred to as sundowning, since their timing seems to coincide with the setting of the sun.

There have been many suggestions as to why this occurs. It may well be much more widespread than we think, since mothers of young children often have similar problems with fractious babies and infants during this same time period.

People suffering a loss or depression also often report feeling worse at this time of day. Theorists guess that the agitation might be caused by a biochemical response to the fading of daylight.

What really matters, however, is not the specific cause—since that cannot be clearly established at this point—but what you can do about it. There are a number of different ways to to help someone during this periodic agitation. Even if the agitation is caused by subtle biochemical changes in the body, there are still many ways to help alleviate the person's feelings.

When someone shows agitation, we can reasonably guess that fear and insecurity are the two prime feelings being expressed. What the person says at this time is not necessarily the actual cause of agitation. This is often when people refer to the themes that obsess them, commonly about one of their primary relationships—their parents, their spouse, or some other major figure in their life, often expressing a sense of loss or anger or anxiety.

"I'm waiting for my mother and my father," says the 88-year-old.

"I want to go home now," says the woman standing in her own home.

Many caregivers more or less ignore such remarks—"Oh, she's just playing that same old tape again!"—but these themes are actually a very important part of the individual's resolution. They often underlie repetitive questions and demands (see "Repetitive Questions"). Wise caregivers find ways to help resolve the issues if possible, since they represent the underlying anxieties that trouble the person with Alzheimer's. It is helpful to listen responsively and offer emotional support. In this way growth and resolution are made possible, even with the memory failure and cognitive limitations typical of Alzheimer's. The resolution comes with the acceptance of unconditional love, and this is certainly the basic relationship of caregiving. The life of the heart does not cease just because the brain is afflicted. However unsatisfactory other primary relationships have been in a person's life, emotional fulfillment can come, with the help of the caregiver.

These themes related to periods of agitation should therefore be acknowledged. However, it will not be productive to concentrate on them during the time of agitation. Rational explanations do not dispel agitation. Telling an 88-year-old who wants her parents that her parents are dead is not useful, nor is it kind. It does not take care of her longing to be cared for as a loving parent cares for a child. It would be kinder to answer, "You really miss your family now," or to ask, "Are you feeling lonely?"

It is more productive to deal with the probable underlying reasons for the agitation. A multipurpose approach is often successful. The likely factors in agitation are:

- tiredness
- hunger
- boredom
- emotional distress due to the day's events
- loneliness
- grief from the losses of old age
- fear caused by awareness that all is not well within
- feeling useless and unwanted

Many people, old and young alike, suffer an energy drop in the late afternoon. Since people with Alzheimer's often need constant activities to occupy them, it is easy to forget that they may also be exhausted by them. After all, these are old people with a serious debilitating illness, an illness that also makes it impossible for them to recognize or articulate their exhaustion. Therefore, the caregiver must be aware of that possibility.

When late-afternoon agitation is a regular event, try several of the following:

- Add an after-lunch nap to the routine. This can also be a welcome opportunity for the caregiver to rest too, perhaps even curling up in the same bed or on the same comfortable sofa.

- If this is not acceptable, try extending morning sleeping hours by encouraging the person to stay in bed longer.

- Offer an energy snack of some kind in midafternoon to help avoid this energy drop, such as fruit and yogurt, fruit juice, or a piece of cake with tea or coffee.

- Give strong emotional support at this time, perhaps by playing a beloved piece of music and sitting with your arm around the person while you both listen together.

- Distract the person from agitation by producing entertainment. Some people enjoy particular videos and will happily watch the same one day after day. Others enjoy the comedy or discussion programs on television in late afternoon. Even if they do not follow them entirely in a cognitive sense, it seems that the energy of the programs is pleasantly entertaining for some impaired people.

- Take a walk together, or go for a drive to some place where you can sit and enjoy the view.

Times of agitation, paradoxically enough, can also be times of great emotional clarity. This may well be the time at which the person with Alzheimer's feels most aware of personal losses. If this is so, do not try to make things right with false consolation.

When we deny someone the chance to express pain and fear, we force the person into terrible loneliness. Do not be afraid to acknowledge the illness and the impairment. You can absolutely assume that it has been noticed! Say something like, "Yes, I know it's hard now that you can't do things like you used to. It's awful to keep forgetting things."

You might add reassuringly, "You know, it's not your fault. You have a physical illness that makes you forget things. A lot of other people have this illness too. It's just one of those hard things that happens sometimes. I'm sorry." Since memory loss is a major feature of this illness, you will have to remind the person of this whenever it seems appropriate.

Do not be afraid to tell a person he or she has an illness that causes forgetfulness. You will be surprised how often it cheers a person up to hear about that illness. Most people with Alzheimer's disease forget they have the disease and therefore blame themselves for being stupid or fear that they are going mad. It is quite a relief to know that there is a reason for what is happening. Be sure to show a lot of affection when these discussions are going on, to reinforce the message that the person is loved exactly as he or she is right now.

Caregivers who have tried the multifaceted approach report finding it successful, so much so that in a number of cases the periods of agitation have actually ceased to occur on a regular basis.

Remember that agitation can be catching. Do not allow yourself to be infected by it. Stay calm within, knowing that it will pass. Speak quietly and persistently to the one who is agitated. Remember that you do not have a duty to take the agitation away. It is only a passing mood and it does no real harm. It will, like most other things, be forgotten. This is the blessing of Alzheimer's disease, as well as its curse.

Apart from sundowning, most other episodes of agitation are reactive; that is, they happen in response to something in the environment—an event, a person, a surprise, a loss, a change. These can be classified as "catastrophic reactions." Look below for that section.

ALCOHOL

Some of the problems of Alzheimer's may be exaggerated through overuse of alcohol. It is also true that the alcoholic is likely to prove to be a more difficult type of Alzheimer's patient. The problem behaviors typical of the alcoholic do not disappear when Alzheimer's takes over. Early Alzheimer symptoms are often masked by or mistaken for alcoholism, especially if the person is self-medicating the emotional pain by drinking. When Rita Hayworth was beginning to manifest Alzheimer's disease, people assumed that she was an alcoholic.

Once the disease has been diagnosed, unfortunately, the patterns of destructive and difficult behavior associated with heavy alcohol use are likely to remain and are increased by the progress of Alzheimer's disease. It is not an enviable task to be a caregiver to an alcoholic who also has Alzheimer's. There can be added problems in that lifelong abuse of alcohol can also lead to dementia in itself, although not to Alzheimer's disease. However, the caregiver's problems and challenges are likely to be similar in the case of alcohol-related dementia.

The most important thing is at least to reduce the amount of alcohol the person drinks. As the Alzheimer's progresses, the alcoholic will be less and less able to manage to buy alcohol, and the caregiver should not supply it instead.   In cases of mild drinking. there may be no reason why a person should not continue unless the alcohol presents a dangerous combination with prescribed medications. Medical advice should be sought. In the case of a couple who have always indulged in heavy drinking together, there is the question of whether continuing this pattern is actually an abuse of the partner with Alzheimer's.

Many caregivers observe that the confusion typical of Alzheimer's may be increased when alcohol is consumed, as can the aggressive behavior. If, as a caregiver, you are going to allow the person with Alzheimer's to drink alcohol, you must observe what effect it has and act cautiously on behalf of the person who is impaired.

ANGER

First, take an honest look at any anger issues you may have around being a caregiver. If you have continuous responsibility for a person with Alzheimer's, you probably get very tired, lonely, and fed up from time to time, and under such circumstances small irritations can lead to feeling a great deal of anger.

If you have a close relative or partner with Alzheimer's, you may have feelings of anger that are really connected with your sense of loss.

It is natural to feel angry that you have to take complete care of someone who used to be a partner but no longer can fulfill the balancing role you once appreciated. It is natural to feel angry that you have to take care of this woman who used to be your mother and now is more like your own child. Not everyone feels angry about such things, but probably most people do at one time or another.

If you never feel angry, perhaps you feel guilty. It might be worth taking a closer look at your emotions if you often feel guilty. Psychologists consider that guilt often masks unacceptable feelings of anger.

Other feelings of anger can also underlie changes in relationship. If, for example, you now have to take care of your mother as if she were your child, when she never really fulfilled your own longing for love when you were little, you are likely to feel very angry. It is hard to give another person the kind of love you never received.

If someone you once admired now behaves in ways that frighten or disgust you because of this illness, you may well feel angry. If you feel overworked, unappreciated, lonely, and never get enough sleep, there is a good chance you also get angry pretty often. It is common for caregivers to feel angry occasionally, often, or even all the time. It is not wrong. A feeling just is.

Unfortunately, anger reduces your ability to be a good caregiver. It is also hard work. It uses up energy you need for other things, like enjoying life. It reduces your ability to feel compassion. It makes you feel guilty too and it takes away your sense of humor altogether. Therefore, you do need to help yourself if you often feel angry. Otherwise, harmful stress will build up to make you feel bad and increase the risk of abuse.

One way to start helping yourself is to become clear about what exactly is making you feel angry. You can even sit down and make a list of all the reasons. That will help you to see what is involved, since there are often multiple factors.

Your first duty is to take care of yourself properly. That includes taking time off, getting enough sleep, finding ways to relax, and getting professional help when it is needed. It is not good enough to say you cannot get help. Usually when people say they cannot get help, what they really mean is that they have not asked. Often this is false pride. Dealing with Alzheimer's is very exhausting and no one can deal with it alone for long without paying a terrible price. It does take some trouble on your part to find the right help, but you must do it and it is really worth the effort.

If you know your anger comes out of stress, you must find relief. In many communities, there are Alzheimer day-care or respite centers to which you can take your person with Alzheimer's and get at least a morning or afternoon off for yourself (see "Day Centers" in Chapter 9). Never assume that your charge could not or would not adapt to being in such a setting.

Actually, day activity centers can be more entertaining and supportive than home life, and they add some appropriate stimulus to a somewhat empty life. Most people do enjoy them, just as most little children eventually enjoy kindergarten or preschool after some tears.

Be prepared to ask friends, relatives, or even members of your church or some similar organization to help with an occasional afternoon duty. Often, the reason people do not offer to help is that they are discouraged by the caregiver—"Oh no, we're fine!"—or because they simply do not know what they could do.

Be really specific about what people can do for you. Ask, "Would you take Mother for a half-hour drive one afternoon next week?" or "Would you sit with George for a couple of hours while I take time off? He likes to be read to."

Most people are afraid of helping only because they are nervous that they will inadvertently do something harmful or hurtful. They just need a little practice and some advice from you.

Join an Alzheimer's support group and start to trade some care with others in the same position. Get counseling if you want help with your inner feelings. Read self-help books and follow the suggestions in them.

All this advice comes in the anger section here for good reason. This is part of looking after yourself so that stress does not make you constantly angry. Another benefit of a support group is that it provides a place where you can safely talk about your feelings and the stresses of caregiving. Do not unload too much on your friends or you wear might them out.

Alzheimer's is uniquely taxing in that the caregiver not only has full responsibility for the physical care of another person, but also has to act as the full-time interpreter of the world around to the person who has the illness. The world of the Alzheimer's sufferer makes very little sense, and it is the caregiver who must find ways to explain, to link, to fill out the missing pieces, and then to supply the emotional support and understanding that is needed. Add to this the fact that many people with Alzheimer's are physically fit and bursting with energy, and the task really becomes taxing. This is why you need to be among those who understand what you are up against.

If you know your anger does not arise only from present circumstances but is rooted in the past, then find someone who will help you work through that old unexpressed rage. If you do not, it will emerge inappropriately. Even if your anger comes from your parent not having taken care of you enough when you were a child, it is useless to take that anger out on the parent who is now too sick to understand or just does not remember any more. It is not fair and, more importantly, it does not help you.

You need to be able to talk over those old unresolved issues with someone who can help you—a therapist, a counselor, a minister, an old friend, a new friend. If you need to talk to someone in a hurry, call a suicide hotline, where you can talk anonymously if you want to. You do not have to be actually suicidal to call. The Alzheimer's Association also has a national hotline and experts who understand your situation.

So much for your anger as a caregiver. Now to the anger of the person with Alzheimer's disease. You hear a lot about it, so much so that you might think everyone who has Alzheimer's also has tremendous attacks of rage. That is not true. Some people never become angry, while others are only occasionally or temporarily angry. This tends to happen in the earlier stages of the disease, when people become aware of their losses and become frightened.

Some people do become violent later, but this is often in reaction to what is happening around them, as well as to them. Often they can be helped by family being prepared to talk about the reality of their situation. All too often, family members decide not to mention the illness, thus condemning the sick person to terrible loneliness.

"I couldn't tell my husband he has Alzheimer's," says Millie, "it would just upset him so much."

There are still many instances of denial, where neither the person with the illness nor family members speak about Alzheimer's. Relatives withhold the truth of diagnosis, mistakenly feeling that this spares the person worry. In fact, nothing is more worrying than wondering what is wrong and why it is steadily getting worse. No one with Alzheimer's disease is unaware of it, whether the name is ever spoken or not.

Many people, on the other hand, never seem to experience the infamous Alzheimer's rage, so do not worry about it. The most important thing to understand is that all anger is based on something that is real to the person with Alzheimer's. The anger is largely reactive, and the caregiver's task is to figure out what the person is reacting to.

Sometimes, sadly, it is anger that has been stifled over the years and that begins to emerge because the person's inhibitions are now reduced. These are the people you sometimes hear about, the mild-mannered man who becomes a raging tyrant. Reports from people working in the field suggest that these people were often angry before but had kept it within. With the encroachment of the disease, they could not stifle their feelings any more.

Typical of this was the long-suffering, self-effacing wife of a powerful business magnate. She became a creature possessed as she plainly showed the early signs of Alzheimer's disease. Her family referred to these episodes as "Mother's nerves," whereas in fact it was her rage at being emotionally neglected for years by her husband who was hard, intolerant, and inattentive. As her illness progressed, it became more and more apparent that she had been deeply unhappy for years.

Such stories are common but they are not really the typical rages of Alzheimer's, which tend to be fierce and short. Dealing with these rages, it is always best to begin by acknowledging the anger. You can usually guess what triggered the anger and can then respond with empathy.

"I know it must be so frustrating when you can't find the words."

"It's infuriating to have to struggle with your clothes like that, isn't it?"

"It really makes me mad too when I get things mixed up."

These comments help by showing that you understand. Sometimes, however, it might be best simply to let the person express the anger. You can make appropriate comments in a calm, soothing voice. That shows you care, that you can accept the anger, that emotional reassurance is there.

There are a variety of other ways to deal with rages:

Distraction. Initiate a new activity, taking the person into another room or out of the house.

105

Car rides. Many people report finding this a useful way to soothe angry or distressed feelings. Being in a car is safe and cozy and the change of scenery is pleasantly entertaining without being demanding.

Surprise tactics. One person had great success using this tactic with her aunt, who was given to tantrums. One day she interrupted a tantrum by suddenly shouting, "Stop!"

Her aunt did so, looking very taken aback. Then her niece remarked mildly, "There, isn't it nice when you stop?"

Another caretaker reported finding a way to overcome her charge's angry reluctance to wear a seat belt in the car. In effect, she took over the job of having the anger. She said, "Yes, I really hate wearing these seat belts. They drive me crazy and I wish they didn't make us wear them," while steadily fastening the device. It seemed to short-circuit the resistance and allowed her to get the seat belt safely snapped into place.

Ignore the anger. This can be done either while remaining with the person or by leaving the room. If you do leave the room—and this can be useful in giving the person the literal space in which to spill out emotions—make it clear why you are leaving and that your absence is not punitive: "I'm going next door for a few minutes now. When you feel ready, I'll be back."

This gives the person privacy for the feelings that need to come out. It also gives you the space in which to gather yourself together. Alzheimer anger can be very invasive, since the person often cannot identify its true origin and therefore blames the caregiver. "You don't give a damn about me!" shouts the woman who really is trying to express her loneliness and fear within the impairing illness that is making her unfamiliar even to herself.

In all circumstances, the first responsibility of the caregiver is to ensure that no harm befalls the person with Alzheimer's. The second is to try not to take the outburst personally, even if personal remarks are made.

It is entirely fitting that someone suffering the great losses and limitations of the disease feels angry. Family may find themselves the target of this anger—accusations of theft, abandonment, hostility, not caring—simply because they are the closest to the person with Alzheimer's. It is only with them that the person can express the real fear and terror that lies within. This does not usually feel like a privilege to caring family members, but in a way it is a compliment. Anger can simply be part of the process of working through acceptance of the illness. As such, family members should try to accept it. However, under no circumstances should the caregiver ever allow physical abuse to happen. Caregivers who firmly state that certain behavior is unacceptable report that the behavior often does in fact cease or become modified so that it is no longer a physical threat.

If you cannot stop the abuse, however, you may have to resort to getting help. Call the police if you feel in danger of being injured by someone you cannot control. Ask your doctor for help with medication if long-term chemical control is needed, but be honest about carefully examining your own interactions and support of the person before calling for medication.

BEHAVIOR PROBLEMS

This category covers any behavior that is inappropriate to the occasion. This includes a wide range of possibilities, from taking out false teeth in public and washing them in a coffee cup to feeding cat food to the squirrels.

People with Alzheimer's do strange things simply because their cognitive powers have been afflicted and they no longer remember what is appropriate on all occasions. Nearly all our social behavior is learned, and therefore it can be unlearned in the course of a brain-impairing disease.

The best way to cope with odd behavior in someone with Alzheimer's is to show the same humor, understanding, and kindness you would with a child. Do not ask why the person did such a thing; it is obvious it was done because social appropriateness has been eroded as a concept. Instead, merely indicate in a non-judgmental manner what you would like the person to do: "It probably isn't such a good idea to wash your teeth in your coffee. Maybe you could pop them back into your mouth right now."

If you feel embarrassed, count to ten and calm yourself before speaking. If you become agitated, so too will the person with Alzheimer's. Strangers are often much kinder and more tolerant than you might fear in your embarrassment. Assume the best. If you feel you must do something to warn others, you could follow the example of one man whose wife had an unusual problem with excess saliva. While walking through a very high-class department store, she spat on a bunch of silk flowers.

He apologized and said with dignity, "My wife isn't well and I'd be glad to pay for those." He was not charged for them. Another man reports that his wife tended to buttonhole strangers and, like the Ancient Mariner, subject them to long, rambling monologues.

He handed them a small card on which was written, "my wife has Alzheimer's disease" to alert them to the basic situation. Almost invariably, people would listen politely to her for a while and gracefully extract themselves as soon as they reasonably could. People often appreciate opportunities to be compassionate and kind.

If others do react badly, remember it is their own fear breaking out. Try to forgive them. They are probably terrified that one day they too might have Alzheimer's disease.

CATASTROPHIC REACTIONS

This means overreaction to an event or stimulus, in the form of anger, fear, anxiety, grief, or some other powerful emotion. It usually happens because the person does not understand what is going on or because he or she experiences a strong emotional feeling about some event.

An 85-year-old woman may weep on hearing that her parents are dead, although they have been dead for many years. Because of her memory loss she had forgotten this and the news comes afresh to her. A man may become terrified while standing under the shower because he no longer cognitively knows that water will come rushing out of it, and the sudden event frightens him. He does not understand what is going on, why the water is pouring out, what he should do about it.

In other situations, overreaction may arise from the way in which the person with Alzheimer's interprets a situation: "I haven't stolen anything. I'm not a thief!" shouts Ruth, entirely out of the blue. Ruth may have been dreaming, or she may have been stirred by a memory, or she may have misheard and misinterpreted something said by another person. She needs to be soothed, comforted, and then, as soon as it seems appropriate, distracted by some other activity.

Sometimes Carlos weeps and berates himself, crying, "I'm useless. I might as well be dead. I'm so stupid!" This tends to happen after he has failed to carry out some task or feels belittled or abandoned.

Other catastrophic reactions may be brought about by caregivers intervening too roughly or too quickly. Never confront, always persuade. Never give orders, always make suggestions. Never push or pull roughly, always guide gently. If you show violence, you will receive violence. You can avoid catastrophic reactions by giving plenty of time for preparations and departures, gently explaining what is going on in a simple way, and never trying to force the situation.

When you try to force someone with Alzheimer's to do something, you are treating that person as an object, not as a human being. You are likely to be taught an unpleasant lesson in return.

Use your imagination compassionately and you will usually understand the basis of a catastrophic reaction. The best way to deal with it is, if possible, to remove the cause. In any case, remain calm, reassuring, and patient. Do not become angry or agitated, since this only makes things worse. Most such reactions are soon over and forgotten. Although they are emotionally powerful at the time, they are not really very significant.

CONFRONTATION

Never waste your energy by trying to confront people with Alzheimer's disease. You will only bring about a catastrophic reaction.

If you are trying to prove them wrong through rational explanation, they will react badly because they have an impaired ability to follow rational thought. They know their feelings and you cannot argue them out of their feelings.

An 88-year-old woman in an Alzheimer's care unit insisted she had to go home to feed her two little boys since they would be home from school. The duty nurse patiently explained that her two little boys were now in their 60s and obviously did not need her to cook their dinners after school. She followed the whole explanation carefully and then said, looking directly at the nurse, "I know what you told me and even if it's true, I can only tell you that in here there are two little boys that need me," patting her heart as she spoke.

Trying to logically prove someone with Alzheimer's wrong only causes frustration and perhaps rage, often for both parties. If you are trying to make the person do something, you will be met by resistance against the pressure you are creating. If you are in a hurry, the person will slow down or even have an accident of incontinence. If you are trying to make the person admit to being impaired, natural resentment will follow.

As in any good people management, the tools to use are persuasion, kindness, and incentive.

If you are being confrontative, ask yourself why. The chances are that you are feeling angry and not really admitting it. Deal with your own anger without trying to make the person with Alzheimer's wrong.

DEHYDRATION

This is a frequent problem among all older people and merits special attention since it causes particular problems in Alzheimer's. Some experts think the thirst mechanism becomes deficient in old age, while others suggest that medications may be responsible. Whatever the cause, dehydration is common. People simply do not drink enough water and do not feel thirsty. Additionally, many older people were never in the habit of drinking water and often dislike it.

For the general maintenance of good hydration, at least four large glasses of water a day are required, and some experts suggest that this figure should be six or even eight. This is apart from tea, coffee, alcohol, soft drinks, or milk, which do not count. Only water counts.

It is especially important to make sure that people with Alzheimer's consume sufficient fluids, since they are unlikely to express a wish for drinks on their own initiative. If they are reluctant to drink large amounts of water, give it to them in little glasses on a regular basis. One or two small glasses per hour throughout the day will ensure they get all the water they need. If they do not like water, add a touch of fruit juice or squeeze some lemon into the water. Try an herbal tea without any caffeine in it, either hot or cold, as another way of getting fluid into them. If the person is reluctant to drink, say "The doctor says you must." That often works.

Confusion increases in people who are dehydrated, so always get fluids into someone who seems to be particularly confused for no known reason. Likewise, give a drink of water at periods of agitation.

There is a quick-check test for dehydration. Pinch the person's skin. If the skin takes a long time to settle into place, that person is dehydrated.

Another clue is constipation. Despite everything that has been claimed for fiber in the diet, the main reason why people are constipated is that they do not drink enough water.

DEPRESSION

This can be a problem both for the caregiver and for the person with Alzheimer's, for obvious reasons. Both face considerable displacement of their previous lives, both may well be feeling lonely and frightened, and both may also be hiding considerable feelings of anger. Depression, as well as being an emotional expression of hopelessness and despair, often conceals anger.

James had been taken, against his will, to a nursing home. He sat in a chair with his face in his lap much of the day, or he covered his face with a scarf. When people asked him why he was doing it, he said, "I wish I were dead. I can't stand this." The visiting psychiatrist decided to put James on antidepressants but, before it could be done, James had managed to die. James's reaction was emotionally valid. He did not want to be there. He was by nature a solitary, unsociable person who only wanted to be left alone.

Much depression among older people is valid, in that it reflects real sorrow and grief at losses. This grief is often hard for caregivers to bear, both at home and in nursing facilities. They tend to want to fix the grief with mood control medication. Before turning to medications, which might have undesirable side effects, it would often be much more humane to try to identify and work with the causes of depression. The likely causes are:

- reaction to the losses caused by the illness
- loneliness
- boredom and lack of interests
- lack of self-esteem
- other losses and stresses in life, such as the loss of a partner or withdrawal of children from a parent's life
- loss of friendship
- underlying feelings of conflict, such as anger or fear

It does not necessarily take a therapist to work some of these things out. A sensitive caregiver is open to dealing with them and often talking about them is the only action needed. It is important to look for openings given by the person with Alzheimer's.

- "Oh, what's the point anyway?"
- "Why should I be bothered?"
- "I might as well be dead."
- "Everybody hates me."

Remarks like these tell you how bad the person is feeling. Allow free expression of feeling and be accepting. Show whose side you are on. When trust has been established between you, try to work on those feelings by talking more about them.

Listen carefully since communication is so hard for the person with Alzheimer's. Never tell someone who is depressed to cheer up or try to change feelings by arguing about them. This approach attacks the person's integrity and denies what is felt to be true. Do not offer treats as bribes to force someone to feel better—it does not work. Encourage the person to talk about what is within. Even a badly impaired person can nevertheless have a sense of inner feelings and want to express them and get support for them.

As a caregiver, never fall into the trap of dismissing depression as part of the illness. The person with Alzheimer's has good reason to be depressed; on the other hand, many people with Alzheimer's are habitually cheerful and upbeat.

One health professional tried the following exercise with a group of women with Alzheimer's, all of whom looked especially depressed one morning. She got them to stand up and shout, "I feel sad!"

They started slowly, not very willingly, but they followed her example. Soon they were shouting with great gusto, "I feel sad," at which point she changed their chorus to "I feel mad!"

Once they had shouted that a few times, they had cheered up considerably. The exercise works well even with one person. Encourage an emphatic up-and-down arm movement to accompany the chant.

If you are caregiver to someone who seems very depressed, it's useful to talk to the person's doctor to find out if any of the medications the person is taking could be contributing to the depression. This is not unusual among older people in general and is a particular danger among people with Alzheimer's because their physiological reactions to medications are notoriously different from those of healthy people.

If you are satisfied that medication is not the cause of depression and you are genuinely anxious about the person's state of mind, it may be time to talk to your doctor about the possibility of antidepressants.

Before you do that, however, you should be aware of two things. One is that you must have a doctor who is both interested and informed about Alzheimer's disease. The second is that few medications that alter states of mind do so without adversely affecting the patient in several other ways. As caregiver, you must get full information on any anticipated adverse effects, and you must also become very observant so that you can quickly become aware of changes due to medication and follow up with further medical consultations.

DOCTORS

It may seem unfair to list doctors under problems, but it is just a reminder that as a caregiver you need access to a really good doctor. A good doctor for someone with Alzheimer's is someone who knows a lot about Alzheimer's and learns more all the time. A good doctor does not treat an old person as if illness is supposed to be the expected lot of old age.

A good doctor does not attribute every health problem in a person with Alzheimer's to the disease itself. Conversely, a good doctor knows that normal symptoms of ill health can be distorted or utterly changed in a person with Alzheimer's and acts with appropriate caution.

A good doctor will treat the Alzheimer's patient with respect. That means asking the patient directly the questions that may afterwards have to be addressed to the caregiver. It means acknowledging the problems a caregiver may have in administering medicine and trying to help the caregiver find innovative solutions. It should also mean that medical appointments are kept promptly by the doctor so that the person with Alzheimer's is not subject to the tensions of waiting.

If you are not satisfied with your doctor, get another one. There are plenty of doctors out there and you pay enough for them, so shop around just as you would with any other high-cost investment. Choose the one who meets your needs and the needs of the person with Alzheimer's best.

Good doctors do not resent time spent in communication and are willing to explain medical facts and prescriptions in language that normal people use. They do not use vague and meaningless phrases like, "She's a bit senile," or "Well, what can you expect at his age?" They behave as if Alzheimer's is the debilitating and challenging disease that it really is for both sufferers and caregivers.

DRIVING

People who have been diagnosed as having Alzheimer's disease should NOT be driving. Opinions vary on this and even official rulings vary. Some states require doctors to report patients they have diagnosed as having the disease to the relevant Department of Motor Vehicles so that they can be retested. Others do not require this.

Even within the world of Alzheimer's, experts disagree. They differ because they feel that patients differ. One person with Alzheimer's may still show excellent driving judgment, another may be very poorly coordinated. In our society, driving is an important mark of freedom. It is often the biggest factor in keeping a sense of independence. To lose the car is lose the ability to manage life.

Recent research reveals that 3 out of 10 people diagnosed with Alzheimer's had been involved in a serious car accident in the previous few months. A further 1 in 10 were said by caregivers to have caused an accident. These are chilling statistics, chilling enough to suggest that no one with Alzheimer's should be driving.

It is hard to lose access to a car when that is what one has been used to. However, it is undoubtedly also true that having Alzheimer's can and does affect judgment in too many ways to maintain safe driving. It not only affects memory, so that people may drive erratically while trying to work out where they are going; it also affects judgment, vision, and the awareness of what proper driving actually is.

Someone with Alzheimer's may drive onto the freeway using the wrong ramp. This has happened more than once, resulting in death for one or more parties. Others with Alzheimer's have driven on the sidewalk or right into buildings. Of the drivers cited to be reviewed for competency by the California DMV, 50 percent have lost their licenses.

As a society, we have to consider the right of everyone to be safe, not just the right of a person with Alzheimer's to maintain personal freedom. Family members often report their own terror at the driving capacity of the person who has Alzheimer's, but at the same time do not want that person to be without transportation.

Sometimes a wife can take over the driving, simply by stating firmly that her husband's driving now worries her. Sometimes families can get their doctor to explain to the patient that driving is no longer possible. One family reports that their doctor told his patient, "Joe, if you won't stop driving your car, I'm not going to see you any more."

In Joe's case, it worked and his wife took over the driving. In other families, the decision to stop someone driving comes very hard. One son actually took his father's car keys and sold the car. His father then bought himself a new vehicle, leaving his son to do the same thing again. It is a problem with no easy solution.

Eventually, everyone who has Alzheimer's reaches a point where driving is no longer possible. Sometimes people voluntarily retire from driving at this point. In other cases, their family members have to fight them. It often seems to be harder for men to give up their right to drive than for women. Unfortunately, their families sometimes see it only as matter between family members, forgetting the danger to others. The question of driving or not driving often has more to do with family relationships than it does with the problem of driving.

Family dynamics—the man whose wife cannot oppose him, the mother whose children want to indulge her—often prolong the issue well into the danger zone of potentially fatal accidents. The dynamics have to be dealt with by the family, sometimes with help from a doctor, social worker, or other professional. The basic issue for the family members should be to keep everyone safe, both the person with Alzheimer's and the child walking across the road or the young man driving on the freeway. Any move to stop all driving should be allied with an alternative transportation plan, to be laid before the family member at the same time he or she is told that driving is no longer possible.

The real question to ask if you are confonted with this issue is, "How will I feel when someone dies because of this person driving, when I knew all along it was time to stop?" That really is the bottom line on letting someone with Alzheimer's drive when impairment makes it no longer safe to do so. Another point well worth considering is that if someone with Alzheimer's has any trauma, such as a car accident, it invariably brings about a decline in general ability to manage and a further stepdown in the course of the Alzheimer's. Therefore, it is not the kindness it may seem to be to let that person continue driving until the inevitable accident occurs.

EATING

Problems with eating can take a number of forms—eating too much, too little, too slowly, or too often.

Most people with Alzheimer's develop an intense hunger for sugar. Sugar imbalance may be part of the cause, as an "overdrive" in the system that demands constant calorific input, with sugar being the most popular item desired.

Many caregivers have no problem monitoring sugar intake. Others find that their charges demand constant ice cream, cookies, and chocolate bars. One man reported that his wife would eat a whole carton of chocolate ice cream bars out of the freezer every day. Certainly there is no point in expecting the person who is sick to regulate his or her demands for food, any more than you would let your three-year-old plan the daily menu. If you cannot hide extra food or cannot deny its existence, do not buy it in the first place. Limit its use to when you go out instead.

On the other hand, as concerned as many of us are about healthy diet these days, we need to ask ourselves what we are saving people for—so they can be physically healthy as their brain deteriorates? As long as someone is not grossly overweight or diabetic, tightly controlled diets are not as important as they once might have been. The typical picture of Alzheimer's is that people gain weight as they grow more ill, exercise less, and indulge their whims; then they lose weight as the illness progresses. You must decide for yourself what your values are on this issue.

A number of people lose interest in food but will eat when it is set before them. We know that people with dementia usually lose their sense of smell. This means that food becomes tasteless to them. You might want to spice food up for them instead of keeping it bland.

"My mother has become very fussy about how her food looks. She wants each kind of food quite separate from the rest and she eats each item separately. First she'll eat all the peas, then all the meat, and so on," Mary said, puzzled by this.

This is common, and presumably it has something to do with Alzheimer patients' perceptions of food on the plate. Whatever it is, just humor the person. If they say they do not want to eat, put food before them without comment. Usually they will eat it. Do not ask what they want; suggest something tactfully: "I could make you a great omelet—you know how you always love that," is much more effective than, "What would you like for dinner?"

Visual-perceptual problems may develop that manifest in strange eating patterns. Hannah eats the whole of one side of her plate of food and then stops. Only if the caregiver turns the plate around will she then eat the other side. We must assume that brain damage may mean she actually sees only one side at a time.

Learn from all good mothers and do not make food a battleground. Eating problems will abound if you do. Anne always says, "I don't want to eat. I'm not hungry," and her daughter used to get into fights with her every mealtime. After an Alzheimer's workshop, she learned to say instead, "Oh well, I'll just leave it there right now, that's okay," and Anne would eat it without fail.

If someone genuinely loses all interest in food, think about serving high-protein shakes instead. That will still supply everything the person needs. A shake does not have to include milk. You could use soy milk, fruit juice, ice cream, yogurt, or non-dairy creamers.

FORGETFULNESS

This, of course, is the essence of Alzheimer's disease, its main warning sign. Until we know someone who has severe memory problems, however, most of us cannot imagine how deeply it cuts through the fabric of life. Our lives as human beings depend upon the fact that our mind weaves together our past and our present to make our future. Once we cannot rely upon our minds to perform the weaving function, everything starts to come apart. Daily life unravels.

In Alzheimer's disease, the short-term memory goes first, followed by the long-term memory, although most people retain some parts of long-term memory to a surprising degree. Effectively, this means that at first the main problems are ones of forgetfulness in daily life, similar to those experienced occasionally by most people. Typically, the difference is that people with Alzheimer's may have less real awareness of their forgetting and things will not come back to them later, as happens to normal people. Eventually, they forget entire days. As one woman wrote in her diary, several years before her diagnosis, "Strange, I do not remember at all what I did yesterday." In this earlier stage, there is also an accompanying loss of cognitive ability, experienced by family members as a vague sense of something being not quite right, without them being able to put their finger on it.

The pattern of forgetfulness varies, probably according to the person's former mind habits. This variation often deceives people at first into thinking that the person with Alzheimer's could remember if he or she chose to do so. Many people retain excellent long-term memory and can tell every detail of their childhood while not knowing who was sitting with them five minutes before. Memory ability can vary literally from day to day, according to how well the person is feeling.

The fact is that Alzheimer's has infinite variations. Crystal cannot remember how to get from one room to the next, but she can play an excellent game of bridge, remembering all the cards that have been played and making correct calls. Frank, who is not sure who his son is, can still play the piano beautifully. So we have to accept that memory goes but that its going produces highly individual behaviors.

It will be apparent to the caregiver what parts of memory are missing and where support is needed. For a while, written notes can be useful reminders to many people; they work to keep some people functional for quite a long time. It can also be useful to label drawers and cupboards to remind someone of where certain necessary things can be found.

The most important thing is to realize that the decline in memory cannot be reversed or stopped by such reminders. Sometimes, caregivers label entire households from top to bottom in an effort to help the person with Alzheimer's. In fact, that is merely confusing. Caregivers must examine the true needs of the person with Alzheimer's and work within that limit.

One example of good use of labeling was the family that put up the following labels in the kitchen. "Cheerios", "milk" and "cat food." Those labels reflected the most important daily needs of the person with Alzheimer's in that household. Another example was the blackboard on which one family wrote a list of each day's happenings.

As mentioned earlier, do not ever test the memory of a person with Alzheimer's. Do not ask, "Do you know who this is?" or "Do you remember me coming last week?" If the answer is no, it is distressing for both parties. Accept that the person probably cannot remember and there is nothing personal in it.

When memory goes, that can also mean we forget the year we are in. The ship of memory can anchor anywhere without us knowing the difference. If someone is living in the memory year of 1932, this is not craziness. It is the logical result of memory loss.

HOARDING

Betty has 22 cans of blackberries stored in her cupboard. She bought them because she liked the picture on the label. Mabel has 53 tissues in her handbag. George hides his money. So far, several hundred dollars have gone missing but no one knows where he has hidden them. Maria, who lives in a nursing home, has 16 stuffed animals jammed into her bedside locker. She "collected" them from other residents' rooms.

Several varieties of hoarding are common to people with Alzheimer's. The most difficult is the hoarding or hiding of money. It is difficult because the money is effectively lost until it can be rediscovered by the caregiver and also because it can lead to accusations of stealing.

Caregivers often mention that they or others are accused of stealing money. These accusations are sometimes classified medically as evidence of paranoia. However, this is really not evidence of paranoia, but the logical result of hiding money and having no memory of having done so. Naturally, under such conditions, it looks to the person with Alzheimer's as if someone else has taken the money.

As a caregiver, you will have to find some workable arrangement around hoarding. A hoarder will not be persuaded to stop hoarding although this tendency may disappear later in the illness. Hoarding is a natural response to fear and insecurity. It is the way in which the person with Alzheimer's is trying to keep the universe under control, particularly in the areas that especially worry the individual. Some worry about money most, and so they will hide it from the potential thieves who are already apparently stealing it. Others worry about food and hide that away. Still others collect particular things that presumably represent security or pleasure to them.

None of us likes to be without money. It represents our independence and our power in the world. Therefore, a workable solution needs to be found that will allow the person to have some money without losing large sums. You might discuss the issue and find an acceptable sum that makes the person feel secure. One woman was content with a $5 bill being left in her purse each day. Another woman was given $300 twice a month. Another man had a pile of play money and did not know the difference. The arrangement will depend on how much the person needs and knows.

It is important for you to accept that if a certain amount of money is going to be hoarded or simply disappear, then that is what will happen. Either the money will turn up later or it will not. In either case, an impaired person is still a human being with certain needs to have access to personal money, even if that allowance is small.

Keeping to the agreement may be hard. For one thing, the person will probably have forgotten that any such agreement has been made. One caregiver's solution was to make an agreement that both she and her charge then signed. In the future, when the woman asked where her money was, they would read over the agreement together, which stated that she would have access to $5 a day, and this usually mollified the woman.

Basically it is better not to argue too much over the issue but to deal with it by saying that no more money is available at that point for some reason. One woman always told her husband, "The bank is closed now," which worked. Money arguments are about power and independence as much as they are about trust, so you may need to find other ways to enhance the individual's selfhood.

Most hoarding comes down to the understanding and acceptance of the caregiver, since hoarders are usually determined and cunning in their pursuit of control of an out-of-control world. Your sense of humor will go far to help you in this situation.

It is important to realize that the other side of hoarding is that the person with Alzheimer's must find things to hoard. This is what often leads to the ransacking and possible removal of other people's possessions. This tendency causes great problems in nursing homes where some patients have dementias and others do not. People with dementias often have no sense of possession. They may claim other people's possessions as their own and guard them fiercely, while showing no wish to safeguard what is theirs.

It is a problem but, as with so many other Alzheimer problems, understandable. They have forgotten what is theirs. They may feel other people's things look like theirs, or they may just want to have them and therefore feel they own them.

There is absolutely no point in scolding someone with Alzheimer's for taking things or hoarding or hiding them. It is a memory problem, not a moral problem. It is cruel and meaningless to berate the person for behavior that cannot be helped. If the hoarded objects are important, like a pair of glasses, then have a pair made that only the caregiver has access to. If possible, encourage the person with Alzheimer's to keep things in certain places where you can find them, but do not expect to train the person to do this reliably. People with Alzheimer's cannot reliably learn anything based upon memory alone.

HYGIENE

Hygiene becomes a problem for a number of people with Alzheimer's, although it is usually troubling to the caregiver rather than to the sick person, who is no longer aware of the slipping of those old well-established habits of cleanliness.

Given that we have many judgments attached to our ideas of cleanliness and hygiene, it is important to remember that the sloppiness or downright self-neglect that sometimes develops is only a disease process. The desire to be clean according to the standards of society is not inbuilt. It is a product of childhood training. Therefore, when disease changes our perceptions and abilities to cope, we forget that training as we forget other things.

Treat the maintainance of cleanliness and hygiene as simply another task with which the person needs help. Do not nag or scold because memory loss has removed that person's former standards. Just deal with it. It is especially important not to scold when incontinence or bowel control is the issue. See the section below on incontinence for a fuller explanation.

Cleanliness is likely to be an issue when a person forgets the old routines of showering and washing, cannot or will not change clothes, and is less able to successfully complete toilet habits. All of these may occur as issues as the disease progresses.

At first, verbal reminders might be enough to keep the habit of bathing in place. These should be as non-accusatory as possible and couched in the form of gentle suggestion, combined with a bribe: "Maybe you'd like to have your shower/bath/wash while I make you some coffee."

This works indefinitely for some people, although it may become increasingly necessary to verbally cue every part of the process, one step at a time: "You could take your clothes off now. That's good. Now maybe you feel like getting into the bath/shower. The water's nice and warm," and so on.

If you use verbal cueing, always remember that the person may not be able to associate words with objects and that you may need to indicate the object you are talking about.

Some people show an actual resistance to bathing and washing, rather than simply forgetting to do it. If this is so, you may have to rethink some of your priorities around this issue. Try to understand the resistance. The whole business of bathing and washing may seem overwhelmingly complex to the person with Alzheimer's. Some people definitely develop a fear of the shower and it is not hard to understand why. These people have forgotten that when they stand under a shower, at some point water will rush out on their heads. There they are, standing peacefully minding their own business when—whoosh!— out comes a violent stream of water. The event is shocking and possibly even unpleasantly stimulating.

If someone is afraid of the shower, try running a warm bath instead. Try adding soap bubbles to make it more appealing. This works well for a lot of people. Or try getting them to sit in the shower on a shower stool, and use a hand-held shower on them. Use the shower head in gentle upward movements, avoiding water on the face, talking reassuringly all the time. If this fails, you might try soaking a towel in hot water and wrapping it round the person's body. This feels good and might lead to more feelings of trust developing that would allow you to continue the washing process.

If you are going to wash the person's hair, avoid running water straight onto the head. Instead, place your hand on the person's hair and let the water run on your hand first. This avoids any shock or unpleasant physical feelings about the process.

Whatever methods you try, some people will remain resistant. They may passively resist or they may strike out. It is really not worth your while to create a battle over this any more than you have to. Cut back your requirements for their bathing. Remember anyway that most older people grew up in times when a bath once a week was considered respectable, with a wash and wipe sufficing for everyday cleansing.

A good bath or shower once a week really is sufficient for cleanliness, provided you can get some daily cooperation on washing. At a very basic level, as long as people wash under their arms, in the crotch, around the anus, and across the face, they have covered all the potentially smelly areas.

Various people report success with a number of approaches. For example, you could get a big container of baby wipes and persuade your charge to use them for self-cleansing after going to the toilet. Instead of making bathing or showering a main issue, you could slip it in elsewhere—as a prelude to eating, for example, or before a visit by a beloved friend or relative. You might also consider getting an aide in to help with this task. Some people resist family members helping with bathing because they feel it is inappropriate, but willingly allow a stranger to help, especially if they think that person is a nurse or medical helper.

One man reports having difficulty with his mother. She felt it was very embarrassing for her son to help her with her bathing and she refused to take off her clothes in front of him. Then he said, "It's all right, Mother, I'm a doctor." He wasn't, but the trick worked. Mother answered, "Oh, that's all right then," and let him help her off with her clothes.

If all else fails, you could try a respite center that includes showers and bathing as part of its routine. Again, strangers might get more cooperation than you do. In the same way, people who hate to have their hair washed might allow it in the context of a hairdresser's shop.

One of the major factors in personal cleanliness is cleaning up after going to the toilet. Many people with Alzheimer's eventually forget to do this. Be sure to have the toilet paper where it is visible and easily accessible. Even so, you may still have to give reminders and perhaps hand out toilet paper. You may even have to be prepared to wipe them yourself if need be. If so, take a good handful of paper and wipe backward, never from the anus forward, since this can introduce infections.

If you are going to regularly clean up the person after toilet use, you should buy thin surgical gloves to keep your own hands clean. They come in big packs like tissue handkerchief packs.

While you may feel this to be humiliating for people with Alzheimer's, the chances are that they will not feel this for themselves. Someone who has gone along far enough to forget to wipe themselves clean has probably also lost the inhibition that made it shameful. In fact, it is no more shameful than needing help with dressing or shopping. It is we who feel it shameful because of the often peculiar attitudes our society has toward elimination and defecation.

If someone is careless with toilet procedure, there will also be a problem of odor and unclean clothing. It is this that people most notice as a process of decline. Try to get clean clothes on your charge every time it is necessary. Carry spare clean underwear with you for a change of clothing away from home.

If the person wants to sleep in soiled clothing, it becomes harder to maintain cleanliness. You will have to be cunning and wait for your opportunity to snatch it away. Some people can only get hold of dirty clothing on the rare occasions they can get their charge into the shower. Others tell the patient it is time to get changed for a special occasion or for a visit to the doctor, whether this is true or not. Yet another caregiver managed to get cooperation by saying she had a new item of clothing for the person to wear. A further suggestion: accidentally-on-purpose spill cold water on the offending clothing and it may be easy to get the person to change, although you might have to cope with a catastrophic reaction.

There is no surefire method. Experiment to see what works. If one helper has particular success getting bathing cooperation from your charge, use that person's assistance as often as possible.

INCONTINENCE

This problem is at the great divide of home care. In fact, incontinence is the most-quoted cause of placement in a nursing facility. Therefore, it is worth looking at this problem in depth.

First, let us be clear about incontinence. The term is used in general to mean loss of bowel or bladder control, but it is often used incorrectly. Someone who has forgotten to go the bathroom because of memory loss is not, strictly speaking, incontinent. If a person does not know where the bathroom is anymore or cannot recognize the correct container for toilet purposes and therefore urinates in a waste basket, that is not incontinence. If a person has become so impaired that he or she cannot recognize the symptoms of needing to urinate or defecate, that is not incontinence. It is dementia.

You may think the distinction does not matter, since the results may be the same. However, the important difference is that someone who is impaired by Alzheimer's does not necessarily become incontinent. Even in nursing homes, as much as 90 percent of residents with Alzheimer's need not be incontinent during the daytime as long as staff regularly take them to the bathroom. The fact that percentages of incontinence are often much higher than 10 percent reflects upon the standard of nursing care.

Home caregivers need to know the heartening news that as many as 90 percent of those with Alzheimer's can remain continent with helpful reminders.

A two-hour schedule is adequate for most people, if there are no actual bowel or bladder problems present. Additionally, always ensure that a bathroom visit is made before leaving home and after getting back. It is not necessary to ask if the person wants to go to the bathroom, especially since this may often evoke the answer, "No, I don't need to." Instead, you will find it useful to suggest it in a positive way: "Okay, why don't we just make a bathroom call before we go out?"

If the person denies needing to, just say, "Oh well, why don't you try anyway? We might be out a while."

This works with most people. However, accidents can always occur. This is where all your tact as a caregiver is needed.

Whatever the cause of the incontinence, never berate, scold, or humiliate the person who suffers it. Adults never want to soil themselves. Someone who cannot control elimination functions adequately is not being naughty or willful. It is part of the disease process. Should you make it a major issue, you will create the stress that leads to loss of control.

It is important to remember that our society itself has some odd attitudes about bodily elimination—hence all the strange ritualistic obsessions about toilet training young children. The fact is that children all over the world eventually learn to control their bladder and bowels when they are physically and emotionally able to do so.

However, in our society incontinence has the triple connotation of being out of control, dirty, and childish. Therefore, we have many warring attitudes within us when it comes to seeing an older person who can no longer exercise these controls. This is why the incontinence factor is major for so many people. One useful thing you could so is to think about it before it ever becomes an issue. Look at ways of coping with it and talk to others who have chosen to deal with it.

Many forms of incontinence clothing are available. You might want to consider what might be most useful. Look at the different kinds of incontinence clothing and adult diapers. If you are not sure which would be suitable, ask your local public nurse to help you decide.

Remember that if you are matter-of-fact about it, so will others. In fact, one man said, "I thought if my wife ever became incontinent, that would be the end of me looking after her. I was sure I couldn't cope with that. When it happened, though, it didn't seem like such a big deal, after all. They have all this special clothing now and it just wasn't the trauma I thought it would be." He kept his wife at home for a year after she became incontinent.

If you are dealing with this problem, remember to keep to the regular schedule of bathroom visits every two hours. You also need to get to know the elimination pattern you are coping with, since many people are regular enough that you can work with their pattern. If someone usually has a bowel movement after breakfast or in the afternoon, you can work with that schedule.

At night, you might reduce liquids to a minimum to try to limit nighttime bedwetting. To reduce your own work, think ahead and waterproof the environment in advance. For example, you can put plastic under the covers on the sofa or easy chair in case of accidents. Also, make the bed with plastic under the bedsheet and, if necessary, fold a thick towel across the area where the person's lower body will be positioned. You do not need to buy expensive special equipment. Use garden-strength plastic garbage bags beneath the bottom sheet and a thick bath towel on the sheet. You might think about using diapers just at night in case of accidents.

You will probably eventually have to take on the duty of bathroom reminders, but you may never have to deal with actual incontinence. If it does happen as part of the disease process, it will probably come about gradually. If someone suddenly becomes incontinent, it is more likely a sign of physical or emotional disturbance. Perhaps the person has developed a bladder infection and cannot tell you. Perhaps the problem is due to a change in medication or to sudden stress. Remember that even someone with Alzheimer's can also get other illnesses or medical conditions that cause incontinence.

Get good medical advice and insist on testing for infections or other medical conditions. Ask if prescribed medications can cause incontinence, and double-check elsewhere if your doctor does not seem involved enough. Just because a person has Alzheimer's does not mean that normal medical procedures should be omitted or that the person is entitled to less medical care.

Lastly, do not worry about incontinence before it happens. It may never happen. Today, with incontinence clothing and a good washing machine, it does not necessarily mean the end of home care if you do not want it to. On the other hand, neither should you force yourself to deal with it if you feel you cannot. It is a very individual decision and you must respect your own limits.

PARANOIA

This is often cited as being one of the problem symptoms of Alzheimer's disease, hence its appearance in this list. However, what might look like paranoia is usually a rational response to living inside the fractured mental abilities brought about by the disease. In other words, it is usually not paranoia but a reasonable fear response, given the limitations of the disease.

"Those people next door came in and stole everything from the kitchen," Suzie tells her son. Anxiously he goes to the kitchen, looks in all the cupboards and finds everything in the same disarray as usual. Nothing missing.

"Does this mean she's crazy?" he asks his support group. The answer is no. Persons with Alzheimer's fairly commonly think others are stealing from them. The memory problems of the disease mean that people cannot recall what they did with their own possessions and that things have disappeared. Often, they misinterpret the world around them. Things are misheard or even mistranslated within the mind. As they become fearful and insecure, their sense of safety is eroded.

It is personal memory that makes us feel safe. Because of our memory, we know our routine, we know who our friends are, we have a general plan and schedule that directs our lives. The person with Alzheimer's has none of these supports, and it is out of this lack that the often-mentioned paranoia arises. We need to be extremely sensitive to these issues within the lives of those with Alzheimer's. With that sensitivity, we can help create a new sense of security.

That said, it is also possible to have both Alzheimer's and a specific mental illness. The two do not exclude each other, but mental illness is paranoia of another color.

PRIVACY

This is a two-edged problem since both the person with Alzheimer's and the caregiver need privacy.

Try to allow the person you are looking after as much privacy as is consistent with comfort. Some people become frightened if left alone even for a few minutes. Be sensitive to any hints that privacy would be enjoyed. If someone sits entirely absorbed in inner thoughts, gazing out of the window at nothing in particular or wandering off into a bedroom, these may be indicators that privacy is wanted.

Tiptoe away while your charge is watching television. Go to your room, but leave the door open so you can hear if anything is needed. Sit and silently read a book.

One of the most energy-destroying things you can do is to spend every minute of the day doing something for the person with Alzheimer's. It consumes both of you and is not necessary.

It is quite another thing for you to get privacy. You might find you are being followed every minute of the day, even to the toilet, by the person who cannot bear to let you out of sight. This is happening because you represent that person's total emotional security. This is likely to be only a passing phase, you will be relieved to know. Meanwhile, you need to cope with it the way mothers cope with similar attachment by young children.

A wise mother would try to work out why her child is insecure and meet the needs for security. You might try the same. Asking questions might not work, since the impaired person might not be able to verbalize feelings or needs, but you can try it.

Then you might try getting the following messages across:

- I understand that life is scary right now.
- I won't leave you.
- You're safe.
- I'll take care of your needs.
- I love you.

Put any of these messages into your own words and keep it simple. Also step up the amount of physical affection and reassurance you give. Hold hands, stroke arms, give backrubs, kiss. Show your affection in a way that is acceptable to the person. Also explain. For example, "I'm going to the bathroom now but I'll be back." Or, "I'm going to put the washing in and I'll be gone for a minute," and so on.

Setting limits is necessary if you are to survive burnout. If it is truly impossible to do that after considerable trial and experimentation, then time off is the only answer. No one lasts for long without private time and private space.

Certain kinds of privacy may be almost impossible. Often, persons with Alzheimer's like to fiddle around amongst other people's possessions. This can be very irritating, but it is only because they do not recognize their own possessions any more. They are not doing it to annoy, but are just curious and all too idle. If you have things you really do not want someone else to meddle with, you must put these objects safely away—for example, in a locked closet.

PSYCHIATRY

Psychiatry unfortunately has little to offer the person with Alzheimer's at this point. Alzheimer's disease is not classified as a mental illness but as an organic disease and is actually a disease of function.

The language of psychiatry is not even helpful on the whole when applied to the world of the person with Alzheimer's. Psychiatrists are rarely called in, other than as dispensers of medications. The use of psychotherapeutic intervention is virtually unexplored as yet in the world of Alzheimer's, although there is a strong likelihood that it could help with people's emotional distress.

The reason it is not helpful to apply psychiatric terms like paranoia, delusion, and depression to human beings with Alzheimer's is that to do so discourages caregivers from really listening to the individual. It encourages dismissal of genuinely felt and soundly based fears and feelings and can suppress relevant response to their unbearable pain.

It is helpful to replace certain frequently used psychiatric terms. Replace:

- paranoia with fear
- combative with angry and scared
- depressed with sad, grieving, or lonely
- delusional with misinterpreting
- agitated with fearful
- compulsive (behavior) with underoccupied
- perseverating with repeating (questions or phrases)
- wandering with walking
- hallucinating with audio or visual misperception

The main reason to replace psychiatric vocabulary with nonmedical terminology is that it puts responsibility for resolving presented problems—such as fear or reactive anger—back where it belongs, on the caregiver.

When psychiatric medicines are used to try to control presented problems by suppression instead of by resolution, it is often destructive for the person with Alzheimer's. Almost all such medications carry heavy penalties for the patient with Alzheimer's in the form of toxicity, confusion, agitation, falling, and increased forgetfulness. This may not apply where there is a dual diagnosis—of both Alzheimer's dementia and, for example, psychosis.

There are rare cases where an individual can genuinely benefit from psychiatric medication intervention, but in most cases medication is given for the sake of the caregiver, not because it helps the person with Alzheimer's.

REPETITIVE QUESTIONS

Repetitive questions are one major reason why people seek help coping with Alzheimer's. There can hardly be anything more likely to drive a caregiver crazy than being asked the same question dozens, scores, or even hundreds of times a day.

You may think there is no solution. After all, the essence of this problem is that the person with Alzheimer's does not recall asking the question nor receiving the answer. Nothing can solve that—or can it? The answer, thank goodness, is that the problem can be solved.

Repetitive questions are a common part of the disease process. The form of the question, however, is very significant. The solution lies in paying close attention to the message beneath the question. The essence of this message is usually the same: the need for reassurance, security, and love. Everyone has an individual version of the question; it is the specific version that gives the clue to its solution, which lies in answering the need beneath the question.

Here are some examples.

"What time is it?" asks Mr. Da Costa, for the eighth time in an hour.

"Can I go home now?" asks Hannah, sitting in her own home.

"Are my mother and father coming home now?" asks 85-year-old Sophie.

When caregivers only answer the literal questions asked, the answer will have to be repeated endlessly. People ask repetitive questions in response to an inner feeling they cannot express, either because they do not recognize it or because they cannot verbalize it. We must look for that feeling, and it is usually not hard to discern. All the feelings that lie beneath repetitive questions really state that this person is lost in the world now. The question usually gives a clue that will reveal the needed answer.

Mr. Da Costa asks what time it is because he is bored and anxious. All the things he used to do are outside his abilities now, and his wife never thinks of asking him to do what little he can. His question is really a statement about how it feels to be stranded in an endless present with nothing to do.

People with Alzheimer's have poor time sense and they are often understimulated. Mr. Da Costa's caregiver could solve this by helping him fill his time. His wife would find relief from hearing that irritating question if she would let him help her—sweep a floor, wash vegetables, wipe a tabletop, do some weeding. He may do none of it very well, but she would get relief from his questions and he would get relief from his consuming boredom.

Hannah asks to go home, even as she sits in her home, because she does not recognize anything around her. Home means familiarity, security, the comfort of routine and habit, of knowing one's place in the world. Because she has Alzheimer's disease, she will never be at home again in the cognitive sense, but she can be helped to feel at home. Her caregiver could deal with this by acknowledging the feeling of loss and strangeness and then offering comfort: "This is your home. You've lived here about ten years but you forget because you have an illness which makes you forget things," says her caregiver, putting an arm around Hannah. "It must feel very frightening sometimes, but I'm here to help you with anything you need. Maybe you'd like a cup of coffee now, would you? And we could watch your favorite television program. It's on about now."

Sophie asks about her parents because they were her primary relationship. She never married and always lived at home.

Although she had a good professional job, she never became emotionally independent. When she feels insecure, she immediately asks about her parents. She too needs love, attention, and something specific to do that can distract her from her feelings of insecurity. Since she always became agitated at night just before dinner, waiting for her parents to come home and eat with her, her caregiver solved this by taking her out to dinner instead.

In looking for the feeling beneath the question, you could ask more questions to elicit what is really bothering the person. Keep trying to find out what the person really wants. If they do not cognitively know, make suggestions. To the bored Mr. Da Costa, you might suggest that the two of you take a walk. For the home-seeking Hannah, an activity that makes her feel comfortable might work, such as playing some music she loves. For Sophie, who wants her parents, you might urge her to talk about them or to look at family photographs.

In trying various solutions, you will find what works much of the time. Keep trying and remember that only you will remember the failures, not the person with Alzheimer's.

Try not to let repetitive questions get to you. Anger will make compassion impossible and your relationship will deteriorate and may turn into blaming the person who is ill for the very symptoms of the illness. Once you become engaged in the mystery of uncovering their real meaning, you will probably find you have more patience for bearing the questions.

SAFETY

"I came back and found my wife had put the sheets in the oven and switched it on," says Henry. "I asked her why she did it and she said she was warming them up—which she certainly was!"

Safety is the biggest worry for many caregivers. It has many aspects—keeping someone from wandering away, avoiding fire hazards, watching the use of appliances, and so on.

It is very important for every person with Alzheimer's to wear some identification. Never assume a person could not walk out of the house and get lost. It does not matter if that has never happened. It only needs to happen once to be a disaster.

Get a Medic-Alert bracelet and have it inscribed with the person's name and phone number and the words "memory impaired." If he or she is ever found wandering and lost, the finder will call the national 800 number on the bracelet or your own phone number. Most people today are familiar with the Medic-Alert system. A bracelet, anklet, or necklace costs $20 and usually takes several weeks to arrive.

Failing that, sew name and phone tags into clothing just as you do for children. You can never assume a person will not become separated from a wallet or handbag, but they are less likely to become separated from their clothing. So, mark the clothing somewhere with identification.

Some local police districts are enlightened enough to have a system like that used in Florence, Oregon, a small coastal town with a large elderly population. There they keep a photograph of the person on file and issue a free identification bracelet. If the police in your district do not have such a program, suggest they start one or ask them to keep a picture on file. Sometimes they will prefer you to keep the photo for use in an emergency. Either way, make sure you do have a clear recent photograph of the person you care for.

Be sure to alert your neighbors too. This is no time for keeping yourself apart from others. Those who have approached their neighbors report getting much help and loving support. Just ask them to let you know if your relative wanders out alone. Often an entire neighborhood becomes a friendly guardian system to help support a family.

Safety in the house means childproofing the house for an adult who has had a lifetime of using all the things that suddenly you do not wish him or her to use. Do not waste your energy on trying to retrain the person. It will probably be hopeless. Instead, put your energy into making your house safe. All stove switches should be off, with the knobs themselves removed if necessary. Gas and electric stoves have one main energy control: use it. Switch the stove off at the main control, and do not ever forget to do it if you are going to leave the person alone in the house.

There is a fireproof hood system that will dump chemicals or sand over a stove fire if pots have been left to burn, but this kind of thing does not come cheap. You may find it easier to get the kind of stove that has a lid that can be lowered to cover all burners. It is tedious to do all this but it is safe.

Remove or immobilize all hazards. If the person is no longer able to regulate the shower, for example, turn down your water-heater temperature so no burning can happen. Think of childproofing and you will get the general idea of what to be careful about.

You may need to deal with the driving hazard too. If you have a recalcitrant family member who will not agree to giving up driving, immobilize the car. If you do not know how, ask your friendly garage mechanic to show you the best way to make a car immobile. Most people with Alzheimer's are no longer functional enough to carry out their own car repairs.

The telephone is not usually a hazard, but it can be a source of problems. Its ringing might distress the person, or it might distress you if, in your absence, the telephone is answered strangely. Turn down the bell and put on an answering machine for when you are not handy. If you find your relative gets disturbed or angry when you talk on the telephone, think about getting an extra extension so you can go into another room and talk privately. Many families report this problem. It is hard to know whether the telephone is too abstract for the patient to understand, or whether it is the lack of attention that agitates. Avoid the confrontation anyway, whatever that problem really is.

Under safety comes medications. Never trust the person with Alzheimer's to take medication in the right quantities. Measure the dose out instead and then put it away. If there is resistance to taking it, suggest the doctor ordered it or that it is vitamins—whatever works. If you think you see adverse reactions to new medications, report them to your doctor. Persons with Alzheimer's are notoriously sensitive to the effects of medicine and disease, so be confident in what you see. If you are disturbed by it, your doctor should be too. If you cannot get the right responses from your doctor, get a new doctor.

The major aspect of house safety is keeping the person under surveillance and natural hazards around the house out of reach. For surveillance, there are a host of door alarms available to warn you if the person leaves the house. Or you may make do simply with a necklace of bells hanging on the door. While the fire department usually does not recommend locking doors from the inside, because of the fire hazard, you may want to limit access to doors out of the house. Use your common sense and be aware of fire hazards. Even a simple slip lock can effectively make it hard for the person with Alzheimer's to figure a way out without being dangerous in case of fire.

SEXUAL INAPPROPRIATENESS

This is less common than people think but it is frequently mentioned by caregivers as something they fear happening.

First, realize that some things which appear sexual are not. Many people with Alzheimer's fiddle with their clothes. This is often because they have too little to do and therefore get fidgety. Conversely, they may also suffer from overstimulation in the brain itself. It is also possible that the clothes are uncomfortable and that soft warm sweats would be much better than the tight shiny polyesters that many older people wear.

Women may undo their blouses or adjust their underclothes without inhibition, and men may undo their trouser zippers. These are not sexual actions nor intended to be provocative. They are simply the result of idly wandering hands. The best solution is to find something for those hands to do. You could give a known fidgeter a set of beads, for example, like the worry beads that Greeks and Turks carry with them.

More rarely, men and sometimes women with Alzheimer's may expose themselves. This too is inadvertent. Their action is socially inappropriate but not actually sexual. Suggest they stop doing it. Often such action is a sign that they wish to go to the bathroom but cannot communicate the need. In some cases, it may even be a sign that there is some genital or urinary discomfort due to infection. If this kind of activity starts suddenly, it needs to be checked out by the doctor.

Occasionally a man with Alzheimer's (less often a woman) will actually make what is clearly a sexual advance, by placing a hand on someone's breast or thigh, for example. In these cases, the correct response is simply to remove the offending hand and explain calmly that this is not acceptable.

The usual social inhibitions against such behavior are being eroded by brain disease. It is not the outrage it would be from a fully cognitive person. It is just the expression of the fact that sexuality still lives as a vital force in that person. In one care home, a 92-year-old woman was renowned for squeezing the thigh of the man who came to do everyone's hair. Since the man was amused rather than outraged, he never said anything to her about it.

SEXUALITY

People do not necessarily lose their sexuality or their capacity to express it until the later stages of Alzheimer's. A married couple may still have a full sexual life together, and an unmarried person can continue affairs with great success.

Some find this shocking. They think that, for example, a man should not want to make love to his impaired wife. Sometimes adult children feel they should prevent an impaired parent from forming a sexual relationship with another adult. This comes out of our general feeling in this society that people who are disabled are not, or should not be, or should not even want to be, sexual beings. Even more so if they are old and disabled.

It is nonsense to think or suggest that people who have disabilities or illnesses should be forbidden to have a sexual life. They may have very satisfactory sexual relationships.

How a married couple work out their sexuality isn't anyone's business but their own. The sexual drive often remains as whole as it formerly was, just as the sense of humor remains whole, the spirituality and the ability to enjoy a number of life's pleasures remain with the person with Alzheimer's. There can indeed be fun after Alzheimer's, and some of it may well be sexual.

The duty of the children of a parent with Alzheimer's extends only as far as ensuring that the parent is not being abused or ill-used. If a parent can form and maintain a relationship to the satisfaction of the two people most involved, the children should be very happy about it. It should not become the occasion for censorship.

A far more frequent problem that arises in families comes when the impaired spouse is placed in full-time care and the other spouse starts to want to establish a relationship with an outside partner. This is a complex matter that basically should be left to the individual concerned. Unfortunately, often the adult children expect the unimpaired spouse to sit alone night after night in an empty house that is no longer a home. Yet those same adult children give little of their own time to the healthy parent. That is a heavy additional burden of loneliness for an already suffering human being to carry.

SLEEP

Sleep problems in Alzheimer's are actually waking problems, the most frequent being the nighttime wakefulness that affects some people.

Often the person with Alzheimer's loses all sense of time. Even though he or she can still read the time on a clock, it does not mean anything cognitively any more. So, when the person wakes up, he or she gets up and dresses and is ready to go out, in spite of the fact that it is pitch-dark and only three in the morning.

This usually happens when considerable impairment has already affected the person, so it will be no use to ask, "Why did you get up?" Pointing out that it is night and therefore time to sleep does not necessarily work either.

The person may get up in the night on impulse through lack of tiredness, because it feels like time to get up, to go to the bathroom, to explore, to get something to eat or drink—for all kinds of reasons. It scarcely matters what the reason is. What matters is what you are going to do about it.

There is no reason why someone cannot wander about the house at night as long as there is no danger in it. The ideal sleepless situation is the night-waker who is content to patter around the bedroom without trying to leave. The worst is the person who wakes you at three in the morning demanding to be taken shopping. The ideal response to that would be to do exactly that, but many of us are not at our best and most cooperative at 3 A.M. In those cases, negotiate the person back to bed if you can. Perhaps a gentle backrub will help, or glass of hot milk and a cookie, or a soothing tape. Sometimes people awake to go to the bathroom and either cannot find it or forget what they wanted and start in on other activities.

The real problem with sleeplessness is not how it affects the person with Alzheimer's—who, after all, can sleep the next day—but how it affects the caregiver. You have to be able to sleep. No one can go long with interrupted nights, especially if there is stressful daytime work to be done.

If possible, get substitute caregivers to sleep overnight so that you can sleep. If that is impossible, you may finally have to resort to sleeping medication for your charge, but be aware that it comes at great cost. There are few satisfactory major sleep medications for people with Alzheimer's. They all have unfortunate side effects, some of which can greatly increase the confusion, agitation, and impairment of the disease.

UNDRESSING

Some people go through a stage of taking off their clothes in public, and this can be understandably hard for caregivers to deal with. It is not hard for people with Alzheimer's to deal with since they have no sense that it is not appropriate.

We can only guess why they do this. Maybe it feels good to be naked, perhaps their clothes are uncomfortable, possibly they are simply expressing some kind of emotional vulnerability, or they simply need something interesting to do.

It is a hard problem to deal with since the urge seems to be quite persistent while it is present. Nursing homes often have dealt with it by either tying people up or drugging them into submission, both of which are extremely questionable in terms of medical ethics and are now illegal in all states.

Some caregivers solve the problem by adapting. They draw the blinds or curtains in the house and let the person be naked. Others get clothes that are hard for the person to remove— long dresses or robes for women, pants fixed up with suspenders at the back for men. It is certainly worth exploring getting sweatpants and tops anyway, since these are soft and comfortable to wear. You might find an all-in-one sweat outfit that would be hard for the person to take off. Some clothing made for the disabled could be useful, the kind that is fastened at the back instead of the front.

You could probably adapt some clothes so that they had

extra zippers and fastenings, some of which you could secure with a tiny padlock or pin.

Not many people seem to want to take their clothes off outside, because they are distracted by their surroundings. If they are inclined to disrobe, keep them moving, keep them eating, keep them occupied doing something until you can get them safely home where they are free to undress in the safety of their own private environment.

If this seems shocking, remember that nudity really is only a social embarrassment (and possibly a minor legal offense). If you have visitors who might be shocked, try confining the person with Alzheimer's to some other room while the visitors are there. Or enlist the help of your visitors by explaining the situation to them, since they are likely to be compassionate and understanding.

WANDERING

"Reward: $10,000 for any information on Walter Harris, aged 82, who wandered away from his home on Friday, July 13. If you see this man, call his son at...."

This is the nightmare of every caregiver and the most common problem mentioned by caregivers. That does not mean it is the most common occurrence in Alzheimer's, since by no means everyone becomes a wanderer. It just means that, when a caregiver does have to deal with wandering, it is seen as a major problem.

It is easy to see why. A person who has Alzheimer's may be unable to find his or her way home and could be missing for days. Others may lack judgment about walking across highways and put themselves in grave physical danger. Either way, when someone with Alzheimer's disappears, whether briefly or for hours or days, it is a tremendous worry for the caregiver.

There are several approaches to this problem, but before we look at them, let us remind ourselves of a truth all too often forgotten: you or I can leave our house anytime we want to and no one will classify us as wanderers. The person with Alzheimer's once had that same freedom to go for a walk anytime, anywhere. That entirely natural freedom is one of the many losses resulting from having the disease.

141

Our problem as caregivers is that we have a custodial role to keep our charges safe. People who go into nursing facilities are often treated as troublemakers when they want to get out of the door, but they are merely trying to exercise a normal human freedom that their illness has now robbed them of. Any sensible person would want to leave a nursing home. It is a warm, cozy prison where you go for no crime except that of getting old or sick and there is no time off, no matter how good you are.

So, let us remember that just as weeds are only plants growing where we do not want them, so wandering is only walking that we do not want to occur.

The first important thing to do is to make sure that if a person with Alzheimer's does wander away, there is some identifying item on the person.

Assuming that identification has been secured, then it is time to deal with the problem of wandering. Most of us get restless when confined to our homes, and persons with Alzheimer's are no exception. They need to get out and about for exercise and stimulation. It is essential that they walk two or three times a day, as long as they can physically manage this.

In the early stages, you may be able to allow your charge considerable freedom to roam if you know that he or she can find the way home. One caregiver reports using a radio-controlled beeper that she fixed on her father's hat when he set off for his lengthy daily walk. If he ever got lost, he could be safely tracked down and brought home. That was an elaborate and expensive solution, but it worked for that family.

Another family managed to convince their mother never to go beyond a certain point at the end of their block. Yet another family were able to arrange for their mother to walk to and fro between two family homes. All of these were satisfactory solutions and met the person's need for exercise and even gave some welcome freedom. It is always possible to trail behind someone who decides to go for a walk and just catch up when you sense that it is time to intervene.

If you need to know when your charge leaves home, use alarms or bells. You may add extra locks to frustrate the wanderer, but this can create anger.

One man reports great success with painting grille-like stripes in front of the door. His wife, with the distorted perception common to Alzheimer's, refuses to step on them because she suspects that they are bars she might fall through. Another family painted a big red STOP sign on the inside of their front door to remind their mother not to leave the house.

Most people are ready for a walk when they want to leave the house. That is why they are trying to leave. Take them for walks and give them that sense of freedom. Sometimes, however, people want to go for walks at inconvenient times, like 2 A.M. Usually this is because their time sense has completely gone and they are no longer cognitively aware that nighttime is not the appropriate time for going out.

If you know they cannot get out of the house and are safe inside it, you can simply let them wander. It does not actually matter if they are wakeful or restless. If you are prepared to do it, you can even take them out shopping in the middle of the night if you have an all-night store near you.

Most people with Alzheimer's who walk a lot do so to calm themselves. It is a practical way to deal with the stress and tension that this disease creates within. Every person who can walk should do so, taking three or four good walks a day. It is good for physical and emotional health and it will be good for you, the caregiver, too. Adapt the walks to the taste of the person. You might walk through museums, through shopping malls, several times around the block, along the beach, or beside nursery schools—whatever works for you both.

Many of your daily problems reduce when you keep your family member busy and occupied. Therefore, make activity plans that help to pass the time pleasantly. If you cannot do this, go to the day activity program in your area or arrange for someone to take over some activities with your family member. You will find it really helps. To learn more, read the activity guide in Chapter 9.

[CHAPTER 8]

Love Works

....

You may not be expecting to find a chapter on love in a care-giving book, but it is here because love is the greatest resource in living with Alzheimer's disease. Apart from all its other difficulties, Alzheimer's usually involves a great crisis of love, both on the part of the person who has the disease and on the part of all those who live with or are involved with it. The person who has Alzheimer's disease has an undisguised yearning for love and is often as open as a child to the longings of the heart. In this sense, we could say that Alzheimer's disease turns into a journey from the mind to the heart.

Typically, people with Alzheimer's express their longings for deep emotional security and unconditional love all the time. Often, we do not choose to hear what they say. Either at home or in care situations, it is typical for these words to be dismissed as the babbling of dementia, but if we stop and listen, we can hear the longings clearly expressed:

"I want to go home."

"I want to see my mother."

"I'm lonely."

"No one ever comes to see me."

These are not just nonsense or meaninglessly repeated complaints. They are the deepest longings of the human being—to be cared for and accepted, to be cherished and pro-tected, to be loved. We are face to face with the profound human hunger for unconditional love. That can make many of us feel uncomfortable or inadequate, especially if we face at the same time our inability to really give love in such a manner.

There are many relationships of conditional love. In fact, they are much more common than those of unconditional love. For example, married love may well depend upon decades-long exchanges between husband and wife. These exchanges are often connected with accepting roles, carrying through perceived duties, finding a basis for gratifications. When one partner can no longer carry through these arrangements, a crisis of love arises. The partner becomes impatient, angry, feels trapped because a certain sense of orderliness has been disrupted and a lifestyle thrown into chaos.

An adult child finds the same problems emerging when a parent has Alzheimer's. The perceived task of a parent is to nurture, to be protective and concerned, to give love to the child, to be unchanging and faithful in the parental role. If that parent should begin instead to ask for nurturing, for protection, for a parental type of love from the child, a crisis of love can come about.

What do we do about it? Often, what family members do is to search for care to be given, instead of dealing with the crisis of love. Either the family member becomes totally involved in personally providing care, or becomes caught up in trying to obtain care in other ways: searching for the right nursing home, the perfect caregiver, even moving to another part of the country because the right kind of care might exist there. Much of this desperate searching is really connected with the fact that a crisis of love has arisen that is not being dealt with. Sometimes it is because a crisis of love has finally been revealed—for example, if a child had still secretly been hoping that a parent would turn into the yearned-for mother or father, Alzheimer's means the end of such dreams.

The person with Alzheimer's disease gives us perfect opportunities to practice unconditional love and compassion. If we can really understand the childlike terrors that awaken an old woman in the night, instead of being impatient with being awakened ourselves, we feel compassion. If we really comprehend the confusion of not knowing what day it is, not knowing a face around us, not recognizing anyone we love, we feel tenderness and protectiveness. When this other human being appears to us unprotected and vulnerable, plainly needing our help, we are touched by that need.

Or so we might hope. The reason we so often fail as caregivers to have this understanding and to feel this compassion is certainly not that we are bad people. Far from it. If we are trying to be caregivers, it is out of our innate goodness. We fail most often because we do not allow the time that love needs. We fill up our day with a thousand different caregiving duties and demands, many of which are frankly not even important, because so often we are avoiding our own inner feelings of pain. We have no sense of proportion about what matters because we forget the importance of love.

If the person you care for died tonight, what would you rather be able to say tomorrow: "Well, at least his clothes got washed so I can bury him in clean ones," or "Thank goodness we sat and held hands together while the sun went down?" The answer probably is obvious when we read the words, but we often tend to lose this perspective.

Alzheimer's gives us unique opportunities to deal with the issues of love—unconditional, compassionate love, unattached to any expectations, duties, or rewards other than the bliss of being in that wonderful flow for a while. None of the conditional love pictures fit. The person with Alzheimer's cannot be your mother if she is living in the memory of being 16 and thinks you are her brother. The woman who is your wife cannot do the washing, cleaning, cooking, and shopping duties with any accuracy with Alzheimer's disease. How then will you find it in yourself to love this person?

One way is to let go of our expectation of the roles that this person used to fill and simply accept the present moment. This is very hard for most of us to do. Without even thinking about it, we are totally attached to the roles we expect people to play. We find it hard to let go of our expectations. Much of our love for someone is attached specifically to that person's particular role. In Alzheimer's, people forget their roles, and those around them find it hard to forgive or accept. Instead, they stay attached to some other time, some other situation, never living in the now.

Yet there is no other reliable moment in Alzheimer's. The past may be forgotten, the future has no reality, but there is here and now. Being loving with someone in the here and now, with no past or future pictures, no conditional behavior pictures, is both very hard and extremely easy. It is hard because we seldom give up our mind-created pictures of what we want from a person or what we expect or how we judge. It is hard because our minds are usually running here, there, and anywhere but in this place called the now. At the same time, it is easy because we only have to sit there and hold hands lovingly and think and be love. It is so little to give, and doing it is like reaching across a great ocean.

A family member may be loving and accepting with a child and yet be unable to accept the same behavior in an adult.

"Yes, I can accept this in my four-year-old, but not in my father-in-law," says Linda. Yet there is no difference between child and father-in-law in their need for love. The difference is in Linda.

Love is both the central crisis of Alzheimer's and the path for spiritual development in the caregiver. This seems particularly fitting because Alzheimer's disease obviously involves a sense of psychospiritual crisis. If the crisis did not exist before— and almost invariably it did—it certainly comes about within the illness. The phrase psychospiritual crisis means that a person is living without inner resources, without a real inward sense of being whole, often exhausted by a lifetime in which few needs have been met. Often the crisis involves early deprivation and loss never resolved. It often comes about in a human being who has never had the chance to become himself or herself, who has been buried in roles and the expectations of others. In a person whose system is already being overwhelmed, as in Alzheimer's disease, a complete dissolution comes about.

We see this again and again in the development of Alzheimer's. Nearly every major manifestation of the disease follows some trauma—accident, loss, another illness, displacement, a fall, mugging, burglary, a car crash, an operation involving general anesthesia. By major manifestation is meant the marked loss of capacity to function in everyday life. Many people get along—falteringly, but they do get along—until some trauma intervenes. Then, family members report, severe Alzheimer's symptoms appear and they are no longer able to get along.

A survey of an Alzheimer care unit in the San Francisco Bay Area revealed that of the 54 patients in the unit, a startlingly high number had been teachers, nurses, social workers, and caregivers. All their lives, these residents had been people whose time had been given to the nurturing of others. A significant number had also undergone lives of considerable crisis and deprivation, especially when they were children. Some were starved and beaten as children, raped, molested, put in concentration camps, orphaned, abandoned. Others had been abused continually as adults, had undergone treatment with psychiatric medications, or had been victims of crimes of violence. The degree of drama in those lives had been markedly high.

Aside from all the genetic and environmental factors that may be involved in this disease, it almost looks as if there is an inner crisis at work of another kind. Just as we now have medically accepted the concept that there is a personality type prone to heart attack and stroke—the hypertensive "Type A" person—and stress-related personality traits linked to cancer, perhaps there is a nurture-hungry yearning group of people who are at increased risk of developing Alzheimer's. Perhaps this is the extra predisposing factor that causes some people to fall victim to Alzheimer's.

Many of us love in a fairly small-scale way—that is to say, we probably love for exchange, for control, for gratifications, out of duty, or out of some inner emptiness that we seek to fill. Loving someone with Alzheimer's unconditionally can introduce us to a much larger way of loving and can put us in touch with an entirely different set of values. We cannot experience that as long we are too frightened to really look at this illness. We cannot do it while we are too angry to be able to sit down and really be with the person. We cannot do it when we are so consumed by what lies within us that we cannot sit still.

If we can practice letting go, being here in the present moment, reaching out with compassion and just letting flow happen, everything gets easier. Caregivers report success with variations of these themes.

This kind of loving is not sentimental, airy-fairy, pie-in-the-heavenly-sky stuff. It is the most practical and rewarding way to get through an Alzheimer day. Using love—real, unconditional love—works. It works better than drugs, shouting at someone, or scolding. It is an efficient way of managing difficult behaviors.

Your doctor might not think of telling you to try unconditional love as a way of dealing with Alzheimer crisis, but as a
caregiver, you will find it works. Instead of fighting to control the
person, you let go and—surprise!—the battle is over. You can get
someone with Alzheimer's to do what you want as soon as you
stop wanting it. It is the tension of the two of you wanting that
keeps the resistance up and, for example, stops your husband
from being able to put his sweater on properly. Your emotional
tension causes confusion and dysfunction in your relative.

If you cannot let go of your mother being your mother, she
will continue to call you "Mother" because she feels the loneliness of you withholding love. Whatever you think you are hiding
inside you will be reflected back by the person with Alzheimer's.
That is what makes Alzheimer's so uncomfortable for others to
be with. Women who were always meek and obedient to their
husbands show their anger. Men who were strong, silent, take-
charge types weep. Those with Alzheimer's often show us part of
ourselves we prefer not to deal with.

If you can relax and lovingly be with someone in the here
and now, you will experience an expansion, a warmth, an
exchange of deep love that will really feed you. Unconditional
love is not a measure, it is a flow. You cannot give it or get it, you
can only be a part of it. When you love a person with
Alzheimer's in this way, clarity and awareness often come to that
person. Again, as hard to believe as this may be, countless numbers of caregivers can attest to this. When you can really love
your mother exactly as she is, she can reemerge and be who she
used to be for a while. It happens all the time.

It is not really hard to understand. We know in general that
even normal people become nervous, agitated, or depressed
around other nervous, agitated, or depressed people. We human
beings do not live as islands, as poet John Donne once reminded
us. We are in constant communications about how we feel,
whether we wish to be or not. If you and your spouse are unhappy, your children will manifest unhappiness too, no matter how
careful you are to be kind to them. The person with Alzheimer's
is not protected by all the barriers that most of us erect against
the things we do not wish to know or see, but is very sensitive to
the feelings of others.

If you are not ready to read or hear this, it is okay to turn the page, but what is here will haunt you anyway. If you do not have it in you yet, you will always feel pinched and small-hearted and echo emptily within. If you can just sit and try some of this, you will experience great changes.

How do you try unconditional love? Sit still and do nothing except be. Look for the yearning for love however it is expressed by that person you know so well. Does the stubborn set of the shoulders tell you this person is frightened to let the need show? Are the eyes questioning and fearful? Is the body rigidly fixed into no-one-can-ever-hurt-me toughness? Is the face an iron mask that hides all feelings? If so, what is the deepest feeling you imagine hiding behind the mask? Where is the child inside who never had enough love, enough care, sometimes even enough food or safety?

Can you see that child? Can you feel compassion for that child at all? Did this person ever tell you about the toughness, the sadness, the disappointments of early life? Can you now forgive everything you never had from this person? If you can, that will heal your own hurts because it allows you to experience unconditional love. Any time you do, it flows back in time to all your wounds and heals them.

If you feel sad when you try this, that would be appropriate. People suffer greatly in this world and our compassion makes us feel sad for them. As we feel sad for them, so we inevitably reflect back to any sadness we have for our own suffering in this life. Most of the suffering you read and hear about in connection with Alzheimer's is not the suffering of the person with the disease. It is the suffering of the family.

"Bill would have hated to be somewhere like this," says his wife, standing in the nursing home where Bill has been put into care. "His sister had Alzheimer's and he always said he'd hate to end up like her."

Actually, at that very moment, Bill was happily walking around trying to organize a group to take part in a musical activity. He was cheerful and upbeat, as he was every day without fail. The Bill who hated the idea of Alzheimer's had been forgotten; this Bill was content and busy with self-appointed fantasy activities that pleased him immensely. His wife suffered every time she came to see him because she was still relating to that gone away Bill. For her, he was endlessly suffering even though in his new reality he was demonstrably happy. Although it sounds harsh to say so, Bill's wife was deluded in her thinking at this point. She was trapped in the past. In that, she was typical of many Alzheimer families.

Until we deal with these issues honestly, we will never create an emotional ability to deal with Alzheimer's. The nationwide inability to do so is killing families, killing caregivers, killing people in the heart, if not also in the body.

If we do not deal with our issues of love and grief around the failures of love, we cannot live with Alzheimer's disease. We are fortunate as caregivers because we get the rare opportunity to practice love every day. We step into that flow as soon as we do the smallest act of love. We can do it any time. Just tuck an arm around your relative or hold a hand, or gently and steadily rub a shoulder and really think your love into that person as you do it. Try consciously letting go of your disappointment and anger and need, even for a moment or two. Breathe it out and let it go instead of holding it tight and pinched inside you. If there are things you want to say, say them:

"I hate it that you have this illness."

"I can't stand it that we can't live the way we used to."

"It's not fair that we can't have our golden years the way we planned."

"I miss you being my mother now that I have to look after you so much."

"You were a lousy father to me but I love you anyway."

Or even, "It's really hard for me to love you when you were such a lousy father."

Say whatever you want to, knowing that it will be completely forgotten by tomorrow and will not be held against you.

If you find it hard to speak so honestly, imagine that this person will be dead tomorrow—which is always possible—and ask yourself, "What would I have wished to have said?" Do not allow yourself to be overtaken by your anger. Speak with compassion and forgiveness. Practice them all the time. Practice stillness. Practice love.

Love works.

CHAPTER 9

"What Shall We Do Next?"— An Activity Guide

....

B oredom is one of the worst problems that affects people with Alzheimer's in daily life. It underlies many of the behavioral problems that trouble caregivers. Since those with Alzheimer's often have plenty of energy but lack the capacity to continue their former activities, they face a constant struggle to find enough ways in that to pass the time. As they depend so much upon caregivers, this becomes the caregiver's battle too. Old habits may not survive, so new ones have to be created. Finding what works is a matter of trial and error.

As a caregiver, you already have many demands upon your time. To also be the source of full-time entertainment can be too much. In this section hyou will find suggestions for a variety of activities to occupy the afflicted family member. It is arranged in alphabetical order for easy reference.

ARTWORK

Art activity is ideal for people who are suffering the verbal and rational thinking impairment typical of Alzheimer's disease. It is also easy to do at home and can take many forms, from buying a coloring book and set of colored pens or pencils, to more elaborate drawing or painting. Some people will reject it as childish but many people will like passing the time this way. If a caregiver can give the time to joining in, the art activity will be even more successful. Clay work is satisfying for many impaired people, as is cutting out shapes or arranging designs.

If you are short of arty ideas, go to a good toy shop and search for ideas there. They will also offer a full selection of non-toxic art supplies available. Many of the art projects that work with young children will also appeal to those with Alzheimer's disease, since—although they certainly do not become like children—they may return to certain primal modes of ability, interest, and pleasure.

BOOKS

Books can be a great source of pleasure even for the person who can no longer read or who seems to have lost interest in reading. Many people with Alzheimer's become apathetic about reading. When actually asked to read something they will do so, but it is almost as if they do not really take in what they read.

They may be affected by brain changes that make it hard for them to comprehend as well as complete the task of reading. It may be that trying to follow a story or plot line is becoming too abstract an idea or is too hard to retain in the failing memory. Even so, people who had the habit of reading may still enjoy the feeling of sitting with a book of their own beside a caregiver who is also reading a book of his or her own. The peaceful normality of such an act often seems very calming.

Even if a person has obviously limited ability to read, it can still be possible to use books extensively. Try getting illustrated books from the library on subjects that have always interested the person—travel pictures for the traveler, animal books for the pet lover, and so on. Looking through such a book together can trigger memories and stories as well as passing time pleasantly in the present.

If adult books become too hard, try material from the juvenile section of the library. Well-illustrated children's books are not usually perceived as being childish by the person with Alzheimer's, and they can provide a lot of enjoyment. Often they encourage the person to read aloud to the caregiver.

Poetry can be very successful, even with people who never enjoyed it before. Its rhythm and cadence is pleasing to many with Alzheimer's. Funny verse is accepted well indeed, since the sense of humor remains unimpaired no matter how severe the stage of the Alzheimer's. If you are not familiar with possible choices of reading matter, ask your librarian, who will undoubtedly be delighted to help.

Some people have tried using books on tape with varied success. Some people are not able to maintain concentration for long enough to follow a story; others love it.

Make use of any story-telling performances in your area. For example, many public libraries have a story hour for children, and impaired people often enjoy this. The material is understandable to them, and usually they greatly enjoy the presence of children. Most librarians are willing for an older impaired person to be present at such readings. Should the older person feel uneasy at being present among children, say that you just wanted a chance to enjoy being with children for a while.

COOKING

This must be a supervised activity, but it can be fun to do. Many people with Alzheimer's can be handy in the kitchen by helping to prepare food. Cutting, chopping, mixing, and stirring are possible activities. Try simple recipes, the type that might be suitable for young children. If you are out of ideas, look at a children's cookbook at your library or local bookstore.

Making cookies is often a great success since the results come out quickly and can be immediately consumed. Simple meals can be prepared together, such as soup and sandwiches or a salad and cold cuts. Obviously, it is necessary to keep an eye on the use of knives and cutters, and people who are combative may not be able to deal with the limitations and frustrations of work in the kitchen.

DANCING

Many people who used to dance can still do it remarkably well even with severe Alzheimer's. It is one of those abilities that seem to stay whole. At home, you can pop on a familiar piece of dance music and take a person for a whirl around the floor. It is fun and, of course, good exercise.

One son who is a full-time caregiver to his mother takes her dancing on Friday evenings. She loves the time out and is a popular partner because she is good at dancing. Since she, like many people with Alzheimer's, has a good fund of small talk, no one has ever seemed to notice her general state of impairment. The exercise also helps reduce her periods of wakefulness during the night. Good dancers are always in demand. It might be possible for you to ask another dancer to take the person with Alzheimer's to a dance at a senior center.

DAY CENTERS

Day-care and respite programs for people with Alzheimer's are one of the best supports available for caregivers. That they tend to be underused suggests that many people do not understand their value, both to the person with Alzheimer's as well as to the caregiver. Many family members simply do not understand what day care is like. Many older people seem to equate taking someone to day care with abandoning them to the workhouse, while younger people have probably never visited either a senior center or a day-care program in their lives. Both need to educate themselves.

"I feel so guilty when I take Mother to the respite program," Gwen says. "But she's much less depressed now and she's willing to get up in the mornings, that wasn't true before. I just wish I felt better about it."

Day care offers people with Alzheimer's what their family members often cannot offer. It provides an interesting daily program of activities much more varied than what is available at home, in a nonjudgmental, caring atmosphere where there is no failure. Family members tend to forget just how much a person with Alzheimer's is reminded every hour of every day that he or she can no longer live a normal life. In a day-care center, it is different. A typical day-care program offers exercise, artwork, cooking, singing, dancing, games, and unconditional love and acceptance from those working there. People can spend time with others dealing with the same problems, in various stages of the illness. They can help each other and share their feelings about things.

Annie and Grace always sit next to each other at the respite program. They can often be seen talking intently together, Annie patting Grace's hand or Grace stroking Annie's hair. Annie says, "So I told them you can't make a monkey out of me," while Grace is saying, "And those flowers out there are just—well, they're—I don't." They may not be involved in coherent dialogue, but they are involved in a supportive relationship with each other. Something good happens for them that is not cognitive but does have emotional power.

It is true that at first many persons with Alzheimer's feel trepidation at entering such a program. They may say they do not want to go or refuse to let their caregiver leave, but these adjustment problems tend to vanish soon in most cases. The period of adjustment is similar to that experienced by a young child entering preschool or kindergarten for the first time. It is often not long before the program becomes a vital part of life. Even though the person may forget where he or she has been during the day, the family can see an improvement in spirits, in involvement in life, and in general attitude.

Caregivers often report that former depression or sleep problems go away when a person becomes part of a regular supportive day-care program. Being busy all day allows the person to get pleasantly tired, thus leading to a full night's sleep. It also helps to restore lost self-esteem and exposes the person to the kind of tension-free atmosphere that is often no longer possible at home.

Good centers encourage family members to stay around to see that all is well and happily give reports on progress or discuss how to manage any problems that arise. Most centers report that the ones who have difficulty in separating are not the people with Alzheimer's but their caregivers. Overworked caregivers often manifest their stress by being unable to let go of the person they look after. They fantasize that the person cannot manage without them, even for an hour or a day. This is nonsense, and it is unhealthy. If that describes you, you need a good rest. Do yourself and the person you look after a favor and help them to enter a good day-care program. Both of you will get time off from each other.

Finding good adult day-care calls for the same kind of investigation you would undertake to find good day care for your child, and the criteria are similar. Look for the following:

- bright, cheerful interior
- reasonable amounts of space
- high ratio of staff to attendees
- well-trained, sensitive staff who treat people with respect, affection, and understanding
- a varied program offering different activities for different levels of ability
- evidence of participants' work on the walls
- display of photographs and biographies of the participants; this tells you that each person is recognized as an individual

(Some of the above cannot be done in centers that provide temporary care.)

It is essential that the center be equipped to deal with wanderers or those who want to leave the building. It is not unusual for people to want to leave a center, especially if they are new to the program. It is a natural reaction. The center should be equipped with doors that have alarms on them so that no one can wander away unseen, or there should be enough staff so that one person can be free to give time to the wanderer who feels an urgent need to get out, go home, or get away.

Ideally, although this is not always possible, there should be a safe walking area outside the building so that wanderers and those who need to walk a lot can do so. This shows that the staff are willing to let some people withdraw from activities if they wish to, thus respecting their individuality.

Centers with no enclosed outside walking area are seriously disadvantaged, since there is nowhere that wanderers can get the sense of freedom that might make them feel less trapped. In such centers, it is especially important that a staff member can devote attention to helping the wanderer feel comfortable. This will probably involve being prepared to walk out for a while with the person while returning to the center is negotiated. Centers where people are physically restrained from leaving tend to have unhappy participants who feel insecure, frightened, and frustrated.

Negatives to beware of include:

- staff who shout at or physically push and pull attendees
- noisy centers (loud rock and roll music, for example, or television cartoons)
- insensitive staff (asking questions like "Do you remember me?" "Can you find your name label today?")
- condescending or infantilizing staff
- too much busyness
- clinical-looking or drab surroundings, that give participants the subliminal message that they are not worth taking trouble for and are not seen as individuals.

Things to check on:

- will staff take the attendee to the bathroom regularly?
- is an attendee allowed to sit out activities?
- how does the staff deal with wanderers?
- do they encourage people to eat for themselves or do they hurry them by feeding them?

Although many centers will cite a set fee that may be outside your budget, ask if they have a sliding scale. Many centers are funded from public foundations and health authorities and are supposed to make their services available for those with lower incomes.

Warn staff about any possible complications in dealing with your person with Alzheimer's. For example, some people with Alzheimer's begin to show prejudices strongly, and it is only fair to let staff know if they might be subject to racial remarks or abuse. Remember, this prejudice is not your fault, and neither will the staff blame the person with Alzheimer's. People who are impaired cannot think rationally and are only expressing their fear when they make prejudiced remarks. If there are special ways to deal with problems, tell the staff so they can make the day-care experience as successful and pleasant as possible for your family member.

Allow time for adjustment. If there are definite signs of distress that have not declined within a month, it may be that day care is not for your person. However, that is rare and usually tends to occur only when the move to day care took place too late for easy adjustment. Most people gain from a day-care program. Their lives become richer and therefore they are happier and better adjusted emotionally.

Even if you are dealing with someone who would never have gone to such a center before Alzheimer's, do not assume it cannot be successful now. Try it first and give it a fair chance, then decide whether to continue. The only person I know of who did not adjust well to day-care experience had spent many years living independently and was also probably too impaired to become part of a group at the late stage of her disease. Many people recover sociability—or even show for the first time in their lives a sociability that had not previously been a part of their daily life. It also gives the caregiver a day off.

DRIVING

This refers to caregiver driving, since people with Alzheimer's should not be driving at all. Many caregivers observe that this is one of the most successful ways of amusing people with Alzheimer's. It is safe, enclosed, and entertaining in an undemanding way, interesting and yet soothing at the same time. Head for a green and peaceful area, such as a suburb with a lot of beautiful gardens. Some people only have the tolerance for a short drive, but other caregivers report that even a whole day trip can be very successful.

Use driving to deal with mood changes and anger, too, since it seems to be soothing for most people. Keep the speed down, since high speeds make many people nervous and sudden stops are frightening for them. For those who do not have cars, riding buses can be just as good. To avoid distressing delays or disruptive events be sure you have the exact fare. Apart from that, a bus ride can be entertaining for both caregiver and the person with Alzheimer's. It allows a time of normalcy and contact with other passengers that can be enjoyable for everyone concerned.

EXERCISE

Exercise is vitally important and too often neglected. Lack of exercise may be one of the biggest factors in wandering in a number of cases. All older people need a good amount of exercise. It is said to be one of the biggest factors in "good" or "bad" aging, and this is still true in cases of Alzheimer's. Since the disease eventually will manifest physical impairment, it is good to encourage the person with Alzheimer's to keep walking and exercising as much as possible (see "Walking" below). Caregivers report various experiences in their search for successful ways of exercising. Some have had success using television or video aerobics, but for many people the pace and the music would be distressing.

Yoga and tai chi are both possible, since they are slow and can be paced to be easy for older impaired people. Others can join in senior exercise classes in senior centers. Persons with Alzheimer's are usually welcome at any senior center as long as their caregiver accompanies them and takes responsibility for them.

When other exercise is limited, it becomes important for a basic range of motion exercises to be included in daily routine.

FINGERWORK

This covers all those small, fidgety tasks that can happily occupy the person with Alzheimer's, coming within the range of possible activities that are useful and produce a better sense of self-esteem. Many of them relate to normal life and can be regarded as variations of household tasks. They could include the following:

- cutting out coupons
- cutting up greeting cards
- chopping vegetables
- folding sheets, towels, pillowcases
- winding balls of yarn
- sorting things

- taking things out of drawers
- polishing shoes or cutlery

All of the above can be deliberately used to engage the attention of someone with Alzheimer's. If you have never tried some of these things, you'll be surprised at how effectively they can occupy a person with Alzheimer's. They are all useful to a certain extent in themselves and this makes an otherwise unoccupied person feel better. Having nothing to do all day and feeling useless make Alzheimer's even more of a prison. Carrying out small helpful tasks lightens that sense of personal worthlessness common to nearly everyone with Alzheimer's. The tasks have the additional attraction of being occupational therapy, and this is why it can be useful for the caregiver to artificially extend the task. Thus, one family caregiver would deliberately carry the towels her mother had folded out of the room, then bring them back in disarray and ask her to fold them again. She said, "I'd happily do it all afternoon as long as she felt useful and kept out of my hair!"

GAMES

Familiar games may still be possible for the person with Alzheimer's. You may have to remind people of games once enjoyed, since they may forget they know them.

You may also introduce new games that are easy to play. Take a look around a good toy store and see what games they have for younger children. A number of these may come within the range of possibility without insulting a person's sense of esteem. There are, for example, many games that involve puttings things together or taking them apart. Jenga is a good game of this type. It is easy yet also absorbing, and everyone enjoys the blocks crashing down.

Puzzles can be good. Building blocks can be fun, as can matching picture games. The visual often works where the verbal does not, so look for games that depend upon the visual and tactile senses.

You can create games by cutting out a number of pictures of people and asking the person to make up stories about them.

Even a verbally impaired person can still make up a good story. One caregiver cut out reproductions of famous works of art, pasted them in an exercise book, and she and a woman with Alzheimer's told stories about them. Whistler's Mother was described as "being worried about something bad, I don't know what, but something anyway!"

GARDENING

People who always loved to garden still get a great deal of comfort out of the emotionally familiar feeling of being out in the garden. Unfortunately, they may no longer be as skilled as they used to be, but it is worth trying to encourage them in their work as much as possible. You might need to actually set them to work, to remind them of the tasks they used to do. Take them out to the garden, put a familiar tool in their hands, and show them what to do. Keep them to the simpler tasks such as weeding, trimming, or raking.

Be prepared for mistakes and just let them be, without reproaches. Maybe you will lose a few seedlings mistaken for weeds, but meanwhile you will have given a great gift to the person, the chance to be normal again doing something comfortable.

If you think your charge might eat the plants, be sure to use only edible ones like pansies, marigolds, and petunias.

HOUSEWORK

"Come on, Jane, come in and help us," called the respite center worker. Jane peered into the kitchen suspiciously.

"Come on what?" she demanded.

"Come on and help me with the washing up."

"No way Jose!" said Jane. "I'm never going in one of those places again. I've done all that stuff I'm going to." It was true, too. At home, Jane no longer cooked, washed dishes, or even went into the kitchen. Her husband thought it was because of her Alzheimer's disease, but the respite center staff wondered.

For those who do want to continue their familiar household tasks, there are many ways to help around the house even when profoundly afflicted with Alzheimer's. A wise caregiver will utilize any such abilities, not because they necessarily make the caregiver's task easier in an obvious sense—in fact, the helping may need supervision from the caregiver. However, it helps the impaired person to feel more useful and therefore improves the sensation of general well-being.

Caregivers would do well to lower their standards in order to let people with Alzheimer's help around the house. The kinds of useful things persons with Alzheimer's can do well are non-linear tasks, such as:

- folding laundry
- wiping kitchen surfaces
- washing up (although this probably won't be well done)
- preparing simple foods (to be done under supervision)
- making beds
- cleaning windows
- washing floors

Of course, if all people with Alzheimer's could do all these things well, every family would want one living with them. In fact, abilities will vary and so will the concentration span of each person. Hilda would carefully sweep all the dust into one neat pile and then, with a dramatic flourish of her brush, would scatter it back all over the room, saying, "There, that is good!"

Various tasks may not be completed and others will be done poorly. Linear, step-by-step tasks may fail completely. Laying a table correctly, for example, is a linear task involving learned behavior and logical thinking, both of that are often impaired in the person with Alzheimer's. The failure to lay a table properly often exasperates caregivers, who feel the person is being deliberately unhelpful. The person is simply unable to complete such a complex thinking task.

Encourage the person to help around the house as much as possible: to carry in the groceries with you, for example; to hold open a garbage bag while you put things in it; to brush the cat; to water a plant; to pile up newspapers. If they fail in their task, do not try to train them. A person with Alzheimer's cannot be trained to develop new habits. Just let it go.

Unfortunately, it is unlikely that major help with the housework will be forthcoming, but try to be grateful for small acts meant to help you. Anything that can help an impaired person to feel more useful is a great gift to that person. The worst thing you can do is say, "Don't worry, I can take of it," and keep the person useless.

HUGGING

This is an extremely important activity and should be indulged in often. It is a wonderful form of communication when other kinds fail. It is effortless, rewarding, and happily addictive. When sitting with your arm around someone who has Alzheimer's, let go of your feeling that it is the other person who needs the hug and allow yourself to relax into the warm feeling of being close to another person. Let go of your responsibilities and enjoy the human contact. Drink in the basic human touch and forget to be a caregiver for a little while. In this way, you will experience that we do not give out hugs, we share them, and loving energy is exchanged.

JIGSAW PUZZLES

Since jigsaw puzzles come in a wide range of complexity, they can provide a considerable amount of amusement. They can be found in everything from multi-thousand-piece giant picture spreads to six-piece wooden blocks designed for children.

Sometimes a little help may be necessary, but encourage the person to do as much as possible without help. When you get down to simple puzzles, you can save money by gluing a picture on a piece of heavy cardboard and cutting out your own simple jigsaw.

MOVIES

Going to the movies can be fun for everyone, impaired or not. However, the caregiver should pick the film carefully. Complex, violent, fast-moving movies cause more distress than entertainment. Think instead of upbeat, human-interest films strong on optimism and easy to follow. If someone has always enjoyed going to the movies, you could try some of the better classics that might feel familiar and reassuring. Cartoons are not usually a good idea, since they are often violent and noisy, and many people with Alzheimer's find them distressing and hard to understand.

If you are thinking of trying out a trip to the movies, go at a quiet time and get seats that are easy to exit from in the dark. Remember that at best many older people cannot see easily in the dark. You might take a flashlight with you. Even if someone has seldom gone to the movies before, it can be a fun experience. Take plenty of munchies and keep physical contact high, so the person feels a friend is right there.

MUSIC

Love of music remains whole even in the deeply afflicted. Singers still sing, musicians often still play if their instrument is actually put in their hands or their hands are put on the instrument. Those who loved to listen to music will still do so. Most people remember clearly the music of childhood and early adulthood and it usually has happy associations. A caregiver can always get some rest by putting on a familiar piece of music and sitting down to relax with the person with Alzheimer's while both listen. Search out appropriate music on the radio, or get some CDs or cassettes so you can instantly play something the person would enjoy. Music soothes bad moods and extends good ones and allows for undemanding companionship. It is relaxing to sit comfortably with your arm around the person as you both enjoy music together.

PETS

The cat arrived out of nowhere, a red stumpy-tailed tomcat with a torn-off ear. Hilda had never had a pet before her Alzheimer's disease, but she and Ginger—as the caregivers named him—hit it off immediately. Together they sat out in the sunshine by the bamboos and Hilda stroked him, saying, "Oh you are such a beautiful little boy—no, not a little boy—a, well, you are—well, never mind, you are beautiful." To the day they parted, Hilda could never remember what kind of animal Ginger was, but she knew their relationship was deeply enjoyable to her.

Pets can be especially rewarding for those with Alzheimer's. They are affectionate, nonverbal, and fun to touch. They have no awareness that their owner has Alzheimer's disease and therefore do not behave differently to them. If you are a caregiver to someone who has never had a pet before, consider whether getting one might introduce a healthy new interest.

Even if someone has never had a pet or expressed liking animals before, pet companionship can be successful for the person with Alzheimer's. A pet calls on the person's protectiveness and therefore creates a sense of power and wholeness that is unfortunately unusual in lives of those with Alzheimer's. For the person who is largely homebound, a pet can provide new interest and entertainment.

If you decide to bring a new pet into the life of someone who has Alzheimer's, it is probably best to bring in an adult animal. Young animals are probably too disruptive for easy acceptance. Adult cats make ideal pets. Animal shelters often have grown-up animals whose owners cannot keep them any longer. One of these would be ideal. So do singing birds, which need even less space and care than a cat. It has been well-documented that pets help the emotional and even physical health of many adults. They can do much to alleviate the loneliness and stress of having Alzheimer's disease.

If you decide to try this, be aware that you will have to care for the animal, but it might ease the burden of looking after the person with Alzheimer's. Make sure to take that person with you to choose the animal, so that a bond can exist from the beginning. Listen to what the person wants and honor those wishes, if possible.

PHOTOGRAPHS

Most people like to look at photographs from time to time. People with Alzheimer's often appreciate having their memories reawakened by seeing pictures of family members. Even quite profoundly afflicted people can turn out to have a good recall of distant times, and looking through an album can be a pleasant way of passing an hour together. When married people look through pictures together, it helps them to recall times they spent happily together. Contrary to what you might think, few people are depressed by such pictures. They do not, on the whole, make contrasts between their situation then and now. They simply enjoy remembering that they had fun or went somewhere interesting.

If no such albums exist, you might think about making one. You can write reminders under each picture. If you are a caregiver who comes from outside the family, it might be necessary to ask for some family cooperation to get relevent information, but it can really be worth the effort. Be sure to involve the person in the activity of choosing the pictures and putting them in an album. Looking at photographs allows a quiet sharing and occupies the time. Remember that memory varies from day to day in someone who has Alzheimer's, so one day might open up a whole store of stories while another draws a blank.

In Alzheimer's there is often a tendency for more distant memories to be clearer, so the person's children may be recognized while more recent grandchildren may or may not be remembered easily. Family members should try not to take this personally, since it is only a reflection of the way in that the memory is constructed and the way in that Alzheimer's destroys it.

Many older people enjoy talking about their own parents and their own young life, and this is equally true for those with Alzheimer's. Give them the chance whenever possible and encourage them in their stories. It is good for them to recall the times when they were fully functioning and could do many more things. Remember to respond positively. If you have heard the stories too many times, get someone else to sit and look through the pictures with them.

SHOPPING

The success of this activity varies. Some people become so distracted by the variety of goods available that the experience is distressing.

Martha cannot see well and she has Alzheimer's disease, so she cannot remember the names of the items she wants nor can she see what they look like. However, she still likes to go shopping, that she largely does by feel and intuition. Her intuition is almost always wrong, and her feeling memory is no better than her cognitive memory. Her caregiver does not enjoy shopping with Martha, but Martha enjoys it, so they continue to shop together for small items. Martha's daughter does the major shopping, without Martha.

Even those who dislike shopping usually love to go into a coffee shop or an ice cream parlor to eat something sweet. Take a window seat so that you can watch people strolling by. It gives you more possibilities for conversation.

SIGHT-SEEING

Brief visits or day trips can be successful and enjoyable for both caregiver and the person with Alzheimer's. However constricted life and understanding may become, many persons with Alzheimer's take great pleasure in stress-free outings. These may include such things as a walk in a park or garden, a drive to a nearby scenic spot, watching children playing in a nursery school, or looking in a pet shop window.

Hilda loves the zoo. She goes once a month, although she always says, "Oh, it has been so many years," every time she gets there. She likes the larger animals, although she does not know their names any more. She especially likes the camels. "They are so—so—gracious," she says.

Since many of the things enjoyed in the past may no longer be enjoyable because of changes in abilities and perceptions, it is worthwhile to try new things. Experimentation is always worthwhile since boredom is often as great a part of caregiving as it is of having Alzheimer's disease. Include rides on buses, boats, and trains, if they can be stress-free. Try picnics in the park, feeding the birds and squirrels, sitting on a bench in the sun, standing outside a nursery school watching children play. If visiting a museum or gallery, keep it short— perhaps half an hour, with a coffee break.

Since caregivers are so often frantic, these outings can also serve to slow them down and bring a little calmness into their lives. The more that the caregiver and the person with Alzheimer's can enjoy together, the more the tension and hardship will decrease. Therefore, finding new ways to pass the time is not an idle luxury, it is a psychic lifesaver.

SOCIAL LIFE

If people still enjoy the company of visitors, or have become more sociable in the course of their illness—people with Alzheimer's often lose the inhibitions that kept them reclusive before—encourage this. Encourage family members or friends to drop by, and be prepared to suggest ways in which they could pass time with the person with Alzheimer's.

Often the main reason that friends and family members do not visit is that they have not been educated in relating to the person who is impaired. If the caregiver suggests something definite for them to do, it helps the visitor to adjust and gives the person with Alzheimer's a realistic focus for the visit.

Possible suggestions to visitors could include:

- taking the person for a walk
- going for a drive
- looking at a photo album
- listening to some favorite music
- having coffee and cake, ice cream, or some other favorite snack
- telling about some recent adventure or happening
- reminiscing about old times, without making this a memory test

The caregiver should also point out the ways in that previous visits were appreciated and how they made a difference. Many people think that because memory has gone, so too therefore has any value in socializing. The caregiver needs to say, "Mother was so relaxed and happy for hours after you came last time," or "He slept well that night after you took him for a walk." Visitors who feel they make a difference, that they are noticed in some lasting way even if they are not cognitively remembered, will keep on coming.

Even people who are deeply impaired can put on an impressive social facade that can be quite deceptive. Sometimes caregivers are annoyed by this. It looks as if the person with Alzheimer's might be faking impairment at other times if he or she can do so well socially. However, it is the social easiness that is being faked—probably at great personal effort and cost. The facade can slip at times, but even those moments can pass almost unnoticed.

Martha eats lunch out with her daughter-in-law every week. One day, the daughter-in-law said quietly to the caregiver, "You know, I could swear that Martha put a spoonful of salt into her coffee. But she just stirred it and drank it as usual and we carried on talking."

The wise caregiver appreciates this capacity to carry a social moment, knowing it is a rare chance for the person with Alzheimer's to feel normal, to seem whole, to recapture for a little while what life used to be like before illness made its claim.

Brief visitors on how to enhance communication with the person who has Alzheimer's. They should be prepared to speak more slowly if they see that comprehension is lacking. They should avoid asking memory questions and they should never speak about the person as if that person were not there.

TELEVISION

Unfortunately, all too many people with Alzheimer's are stuck in front of a television nearly all day, that is destructive of their capacity to function. However, the judicious use of television can be fun.

You will have to find out by experimentation what really works. Many people enjoy soap operas, even if they do not follow the action closely. Others like talk shows, especially if they are mildly shocking.

Other good possibilities include:

- "Wheel of Fortune" (a universal favorite of people with Alzheimer's, for some reason)
- "Sesame Street"
- good-natured comedy shows
- nature programs

- movie classics
- musical programs

  Programs to avoid might include:

- news
- cartoons, that tend to be noisy, violent, and confusing
- violent, fast-moving programs
- distressing, bloody, or noisy programs

If you find that someone has a favorite program or film, you can read on your VCR and keep it for a mood-fixer when that person needs cheering or amusing.

TOYS

All of us have our toys—although we may not always think of them in that way— and so too should the person with Alzheimer's.

To find the ideal toy takes time and experimentation, together with sensitivity. People who have Alzheimer's do not forget that they hate being treated like children. If they clearly identify a toy as being meant for a child, they will tend to reject it.

Many toys, however, cross the child/adult boundaries. Furry animals are often very acceptable, because they are soft and comforting to have around. Other suitable toys might include:

- simple puzzles
- objects pleasing for their feel, such as foam rubber toys, wooly toys, anything soft
- simple construction kits
- bubble-blowing solution
- big soft balls
- colored paper to cut up
- coloring books
- colored stones

Many of the toys that appeal to children aged two to five may come within the range of severely impaired adults and prove to be amusing and pleasant to pass the time with. However, it is important to recognize that while these toys are used by children as learning and growth tools, they are simply a source of amusement to the person with Alzheimer's. They should not be used to try to train a memory-impaired person, since this will only cause stress and uneasiness.

A toy is good enough if it helps to bring activity and mild challenge to an understimulated person. It may never improve the person's condition but at least it may keep boredom and depression at bay. A person who is undernourished with activity will decline quickly.

WALKING

This is a necessary activity for people with Alzheimer's unless they are so physically impaired that it is impossible. It is an easy form of exercise and yet supplies much of the stimulus needed to keep the body in good working order. It helps to bring healthy tiredness and may enable someone to sleep much better. It may also cut down the wandering that can be such a problem to caregivers.

People with Alzheimer's who can express their inner feelings talk of the severe depression and uneasiness that can be controlled and evaporated through the physically soothing act of walking. Walking is necessary for calmness and peace of mind. In fact, recent studies have demonstrated that people with Alzheimer's who walk regularly every day actually do better in maintaining cognitive functioning than those who are encouraged to talk but not specifically engaged in walking. From this we can see that walking is not merely a pleasant pastime but is essential to the person's well-being.

Comfortable shoes are a must for this. Good sneakers might be best, since they are strong, soft, and supportive and leave room for warm socks to be worn. Persons with Alzheimer's are very sensitive to wind, cold, and rain. They may experience them as feeling extremely uncomfortable or as overstimulating. If they want to wrap up warmly, even on a summer day, let them.

The body's thermostat definitely gets deranged by dementia and many people become upset by even mildly unpleasant weather. Do not fight over clothing, just be prepared to carry it if it gets to be too much for the person.

Many people become less coordinated snd less physically able as their Alzheimer's disease progresses, but it is still important to encourage them to take daily walks if possible. Frequent rests may be needed.

"Help, I'm Going Crazy!"— Caring for the Caregiver

··

> *"I know I'm under stress. And it isn't fair to Bill. It's not his fault he's sick, but I find myself screaming at him sometimes. Once I made him cry. You can't imagine what I felt like, watching that big strong man standing there with tears running down his face. I cried too and I said, 'I'm sorry but it's so hard looking after you.' He didn't say anything, just looked sad."*
>
> —ELLIE, age 59, whose husband Bill, age 67, has Alzheimer's disease

Looking after a person who has Alzheimer's disease is exceptionally demanding. The dementias are more demanding than obviously physical illnesses like cancer. Because people with Alzheimer's can look surprisingly well and fit, we are often deceived by this appearance. Because they look fine, caregivers tend to subconsciously make the assumption that they are fine—despite all the evidence to the contrary. Then the caregivers wonder why they cannot cope with the demands of caring for someone who appears well.

If the person with Alzheimer's looked as ill as the person in a comparable stage of cancer, we would clearly see how advanced the illness was. Someone with terminal cancer tends to look thin, often yellowish or livid white, and may be largely bedridden. Visible warnings remind us daily how ill the person is, and that reminder tempers our behavior and understanding.

174

However, a person with middle- or late-stage Alzheimer's may look well. This often deceives caregivers into blaming themselves for not being better at looking after this person. The person may appear cheerful, physically in good condition, able to walk about freely, full of energy. Seeing that deceptively hale appearance, it is hard to remember how ill this person really is. It is even more difficult when outsiders reinforce this: "Fred looks so good, doesn't he? It's hard to believe he's as bad as you say." "I talked to Mom on the phone the other day and she sounded great. Just like old times. Are you sure she's got Alzheimer's?" Friends and relatives mean no malice by remarks like this, but they make caregivers inwardly reproach themselves even more for their failures.

It is more useful to compare the average family caregiver with the hired professional. If you wanted a registered nurse to look after your severely impaired mother, for a start you would be forced to hire a nurse for each of three eight-hour shifts. This alone tells you how much attention the person with Alzheimer's needs.

As any family caregiver knows, looking after someone with Alzheimer"s is a 24-hour task. Constant supervision, day and night, is essential. Unbroken sleep may be impossible. As well as taking over all the normal personal care and household chores, you will also probably have to help that person with every task of daily life, including dressing, washing, and going to the bathroom.

As if that were not enough, you will probably also have to keep explaining the world to the person, filling the sense gaps that are missing, soothing and calming. You may well have to repeat your answers dozens, scores, or hundreds of times a day—and you will be unable to rely on that person's remembering one single comment, answer, or instruction you gave. Instead, you will be fully employed as a 24-hour interpreter, ready at any time of day or night to make the connections they cannot.

Who on earth could do all that? The answer, unfortunately, is that the average family caregiver drives himself or herself to try. That is why the Alzheimer's Association reports that over 66 percent of home caregivers suffer from emotional, physical, or mental illness due to the stress of caregiving. When elderly spouses are concerned, it is not uncommon for the well spouses to work themselves into the grave while their partners with Alzheimer's are still going strong.

STOP!

Stop now and take a hard look at what you have to do. Make a list of your daily tasks—all of them—from the practical assistance to the number of hours you have to remain constantly alert. Take account of the few uninterrupted hours of sleep you can rely upon getting. Make another list of the things you worry about. Add any concerns you have about your own health. Now make separate list of all the things you do to look after yourself. If that particular list is empty—and unfortunately it may well be—it is time to reevaluate.

You must not go on endlessly coping alone. The price of doing that includes heart attacks, strokes, ulcers, and other catastrophic illnesses—and that is the good news. That assumes you will survive at all. Many people do not. They try so hard to look after someone—for example, a spouse—that they die and leave their spouse alone. Alzheimer's cannot be coped with alone. It is self-destructive even to try. It makes no sense.

Like many people, you may have been brought up to believe that, whatever your troubles were, you dealt with them yourself. You did not ask others for help and you did not let anyone outside the family even know about your problems. None of this can apply to dealing with Alzheimer's. No one can deal with it alone. You must reach out to others for help. You have to get involved beyond your family if you are to get the support you need, in order to survive the stress of caregiving. You have to become willing to ask for what you need instead of being private and concealing.

"I was ashamed of Claire when she got Alzheimer's. I got mad at her because she did strange things. If she did them in public, I felt like hitting her. She had a daughter but she never helped me with her mother. It was just me, and I'm afraid I wasn't very patient," says Virgil, whose wife Claire is now in a care home, after he was hospitalized with a stroke.

Perhaps you think you are not stressed, that you are managing well. Check out the following list of stress indicators:

- muscle tightness, neck, back, and shoulder aches

- dragging headaches that never go away
- inability to sleep, waking in the night, and being unable to get back to sleep, waking at dawn and lying sleepless for hours
- pains that wander around the body, disappearing from one place only to appear in another
- stomach, digestive, gastrointestinal problems without real physical cause
- destlessness so that even if you get a chance to rest and relax, you cannot do so
- gritting or grinding your teeth
- numerous small accidents
- inability to concentrate
- mood swings, flying off the handle, weeping fits
- increased outbreaks of arthritis, bursitis, and any other -itis
- increased reliance upon alcohol to relax, pills to sleep, tranquilizers to calm down
- decreased socialization
- fear of others, "can't-be-botheredness" about others, blaming others for everything
- palpitations or chest pains not due to angina or heart trouble
- inability to carry out the normal tasks of life
- increased forgetfulness, so that you worry about whether you might have Alzheimer's yourself
- watching television for hours every day, even when you are not actually interested in the programs
- having a feeling of despair, being overwhelmed, depressed, overanxious

The list could go on for pages, since human beings manifest distress in hundreds of different ways. However, if you can tick off several of the items on the list, then believe it: You are suffering from stress. And stress kills.

One of the best ways for you to begin dealing with the stress of being a caregiver is to make contact with other caregivers.

"It took me far too long to join a support group," says Jean. "I should have joined as soon as I started taking care of my mother, but I said to myself, 'I'm a nurse. I know how to take care of people. It's my profession.' But it's different when it's your own mother or spouse. You need to be able to talk things over with other people who really know what it's like."

Most of those caregivers who find their way to a support group find it enormously helpful. It is a great pity that so many people doubt the usefulness of such groups.

"What's the use of getting together with a bunch of people feeling sorry for themselves?" says Al. "You'd just feel worse afterwards, wouldn't you?"

Many families seek the help of support groups because they feel abandoned in their struggle with Alzheimer's. It is not, as you might fear, just a bunch of people complaining to each other. It is a group of people who sometimes complain—certainly—but who give each other good information, have a whole range of suggestions for coping with problems, who represent among themselves a wide range of experience, knowledge, and ideas for dealing with Alzheimer's. Support group members have access to the experience of Alzheimer's in a way that no medical professional, no social worker—no one who does not actually live with the disease—can share. They can recommend a good doctor, a particularly helpful social worker, or a great daycare program. They can also ease your burden simply by knowing how you feel without your having to explain.

"I got Edie up three times yesterday, got her dressed, and each time when I came back, she was back under the covers undressed again. I could have killed her," says Wayne. The group nods feelingly. They have all known those moments of frustration. "Sometimes I fantasize about putting her out on the freeway just when an 18-wheeler is coming along." The group laughs, because they understand exactly how Wayne feels and they know he is only partly joking. When he gets home, Wayne feels better just because he has not been alone and because he could tell these people his secrets and not be condemned by them.

Remember that support groups differ in their personality, varying with the members as well as the individual facilitator. If you do not like the first one you go to, another one might be perfect for you. Most areas have at least two groups to choose from; large metropolitan areas tend to have a wide selection.

Find a support group through the Alzheimer's Association national number (1-800-621-0379 for all states other than Illinois; within Illinois, 1-800-572-6037), or check the local senior or social services agency. Groups are also listed in most local newspapers or at the public library.

Most Alzheimer's support groups in this country are sponsored by the national Alzheimer's Association, which does the supremely helpful task of putting out information and newsletters, as well as organizing training and workshops, in addition to national advocacy and fund-raising for research into the cause, treatment, and cure of Alzheimer's disease. All Alzheimer's Association groups are free of charge. Their facilitators are unpaid volunteers who are usually highly knowledgeable about living with Alzheimer's disease.

You may also find other free support groups, perhaps organized through your local hospital as a community service or as part of a local day respite program. Some groups might be for all home caregivers, not Alzheimer-specific. If this is all that is available, you would probably find it useful. Most Alzheimer and dementia caregivers find specific groups more helpful, but all full-time caregiving is equally troublesome and therefore all caregivers can help each other.

However overstressed you are right now, you can immediately begin to change the way in which you are living your life. The first step in doing this is to recognize that you have a supreme responsibility to take care of yourself first. If you do not take care of yourself, you cannot be a good caregiver. If you do not take steps to deal with your stress, then your stress will deal with you. It does not feel very natural to put yourself first when you have been used to looking after someone else and putting that other person first.

"Fred and I used to play bingo on Mondays and he doesn't want to do it now. He tells me to go by myself but I feel so guilty about leaving him behind," says Laura to her support group.

"Would you leave him alone?" asks Eva.

"Of course not!" Laura looks shocked. "My son says he'd stay with him."

The group encourages her to try an evening by herself. The following month she confesses she has done so. She enjoyed herself and Fred had not missed her.

It may feel selfish or just plain impossible, or you may not know how to put yourself first. After all, you still have that other person totally needing your care. How could you possibly put yourself first? This often unanswered question is the center of the Alzheimer caregiver's real problem. It is not that caregiving in itself has to be so stressful. It is that disregarding one's own needs causes the stress. Caregiving need not be a totally unrewarding and self-punitive experience. We have a lot of leeway in changing aspects of our life that lead to stress.

"I kept telling myself I could take time for me when Sam was dead. But it's been five years now and this year the doctor said my stomach pains were due to an ulcer. He said if I didn't stop, Sam would outlive me anyway," Rachel says.

Her doctor recommended medication for her ulcer and a therapist for her stress. "The therapist helped me to see that all my problems were not due to Sam's Alzheimer's, but partly to do with how I coped. I kept thinking I couldn't possibly feel better until his Alzheimer's was solved. She helped me see I could feel better right now if I dealt with my stress."

Rachel has not changed her routine radically, but she has made changes that help her refocus. She takes soothing baths with healing oils. She goes to a movie once a week by herself. She gets up earlier so she can have an hour of peace in the morning before Sam awakes.

"Sam's as ill as ever but I'm doing better," she says.

You can do better too by acknowledging that you do need help from outside and planning your campaign for obtaining it. Take each day and its obligations and make a list of them. Then assess how you can get more help. If you do not sleep through the night, can you get a relative to relieve you of your nighttime duties? Can you afford help in the house? Perhaps a live-in student could carry some duties in return for room, board, and perhaps a small salary. Have you looked into the day-care programs in your area? Do you know where local respite centers are? Perhaps you can sleep in the daytime or go to bed earlier or find other ways to change your routine that would help you. You might have to struggle to be flexible.

Louella looked after her brother who had dementia, not medically diagnosed. After a couple of years of looking after him, he became less able to walk. It would have been easier to manage if she had changed her downstairs sewing room into his bedroom and moved her sewing room upstairs. However, Louella felt it was not respectable for him to have a bedroom downstairs next to the kitchen. She had to all but drag him upstairs every night and then back downstairs in the morning, since she could not trust him alone. They went on like this until her brother fell on the stairs, broke a hip, and was placed in a nursing home. Louella felt bad about it but she was unable to adapt to the reality of his situation.

Getting assistance also means asking family members to give more practical help and being very specific about what, when, why, and how they will help. Often, family members resist vaguer suggestions because you allow them space to evade your request. "I wish you would help more" is likely to bring the answer, "Oh yes, well, I'll try," and no actual practical contribution. You might get more results if you state exactly what you want.

It is harder for a family member to evade when you say, "I want to go to that painting class I told you about. Will you come over on Wednesday evenings and sit with your father, please?" At least, such a direct question tells you exactly what you are up against if you get the answer "no".

If you can, avoid reproach, whining, or martyrdom when you tell your family what you need. It is easy for them to turn you off if you generalize about your difficulties. Instead, be direct and ask for precise commitments from them. The same is true with friends and neighbors. Unfortunately, you cannot always count on your friends to be around when Alzheimer's strikes. Joanne's story is typical.

"Our friends just slowly disappeared when Harold got Alzheimer's," she recalls. These weren't casual friends. They were two or three couples we had known for years—gone on holiday with them, spent Thanksgiving and Christmas with them. Gradually they were no longer around and we stopped getting invitations. I can't tell you how much that hurt me. The sorrow is even greater than the loneliness I feel. How could they do that to us?"

We all know that some friends are better than others in times of trouble. In fact, some people are actually better friends when we are in trouble than when life is going smoothly. That is no reflection on anyone. People have different coping skills, and the nearer a problem gets to their own fear level, the further away they are likely to be—unless they are emotionally mature people. Being older, alas, is no guarantee of emotional maturity. Alzheimer's strikes at the very heart of most people's fear center. Since there is so much Alzheimer's around without known cause, many people fear it.

Those who dread Alzheimer's fear that it means loss, dependency on others, lack of freedom, perhaps lack of dignity, not being able to count on oneself any more. The older people get, the more they fear this disease they hear so much about. When someone they know and love, someone who has been as competent as themselves, is diagnosed as having it, many people run.

On the other hand, not everyone behaves like this. When Mike found that his wife had Alzheimer's, he called together 12 of their closest friends for a meeting. "Mabel has Alzheimer's disease," he began. "I know you'll all be sorry to hear that and I know it might make some of you want to avoid us. I'll understand if you do that, but I sure will miss you and so will Mabel."

That gave his friends an unusual opportunity, to discuss together with each other's support their own feelings and fears about Alzheimer's. After a while, Mike continued:

"Now here's what we're going to need. I have to stay up nights pretty often now since Mabel gets up and wanders about. So if any of you could come over in the mornings sometimes, so I could catch up a bit on my sleep, why that'd be just dandy. And you know I still like to fish, so if any of you ladies would take Mabel out for coffee or home for lunch so I can get a break that way, well, that'd be just great too."

One by one, he told his friends what he needed and how much he and Mabel still wanted their friends' love and help and company. At last report, Mike said they'd only lost one couple from their social group. The others were chipping in with help and relief whenever they could and they still invited Mike and Mabel over, accepting that Mike could not return their hospitality the same way. (He never has learned to be a really good cook like Mabel was.)

That is a rare success story but probably not because such friends are rare. More likely, the rarity was Mike's courage and honesty in putting out his needs and the risk he took in really reaching out to his friends. Not many people are as brave as Mike. It is much more usual for people to say, "There's no help out there," rather than learn how to ask for it in the right way. It is probably part of the older generation's pride that says one must cope alone, but it also represents shrinking away from the risk of possible refusal. It takes real courage to ask, and it is true there is no guarantee of success. One woman had been encouraged by her support group to ask a friend to take her mother out occasionally. Later she reported back to the group: "I asked Mother's friend Sallie if she'd help me by taking Mother for a drive. She said she couldn't possibly have that much responsibility for her!"

So, there is a personal risk in asking. Set against the much higher risk—or even the certainty—of failing in the task of being a good caregiver if you do not ask, it will be better in the long run to ask people for what you need. In the same way, make sure your neighbors know about your family member's condition. That way, they will become part of your defense system. Few people are unneighborly about such things. In general, people like to help if they know how they can and feel confident about it. Often they hesitate only because they are not sure if they would be welcome in their intervention, and they may fear they will hurt or upset the person with Alzheimer's if they do not always know exactly how to deal with them.

"I think our neighbor's husband has Alzheimer's. He has that kind of lost look about him," Phyllis says. "I've tried to make conversation with her, so I could offer some help, but she won't talk to me apart from saying hello. Poor thing, she looks so tired. I'd like to help but..." Phyllis shrugs. Being open to accepting help from others will enable you to look after yourself better.

How else will you look after yourself? One major way you can help your stress is to come to terms with what is going on. Human beings often get entangled in their problems and tend to tell themselves, "I can't expect to feel better until this problem is over." So the caregiver may be saying inside, "There's no relief for me until he [or she] is dead." Thinking this may well be creating even more stress because of the guilt that such secret thoughts often cause. Actually, such thoughts are totally normal. Even the most loving caregiver thinks, sometimes sadly and sometimes longingly, of being released from a burden by the death of the person with Alzheimer's.

It is true there will be problems and situations to be dealt with until death does occur. However, the stress of dealing with the situation can be alleviated at any moment by the actions we take. This is such a simple way to help ourselves that hardly anyone ever does so. We tend to think in terms of big, impossible solutions for our biggest problems, but we could find it very helpful to think smaller. The Chinese say: "If you can't change a situation, you must change your mind."

You can deal with the results of stress right now. You can sit down and take ten slow, deep breaths. And you can do this several times a day every day—especially before you sleep, when you get up, and during any particularly stressful time. You can do some basic stretching exercises to help your muscle tension. You can soak in a hot scented tub for a while. You can buy a bunch of flowers and look at them with enjoyment. You can write down a list of everything that is worrying you and cross off all items you cannot do anything about here and now. You can stop fighting the fact of Alzheimer's and accept that it is here and it will have certain effects on the person who has it.

You can look into stress management classes at your local senior center or community college. You can learn how to deal with tension, headaches, and other bodily symptoms. You can take up meditation, self-hypnosis, relaxation. Actually, you undoubtedly already know many of the ways you could instantly reduce your stress. The trick is to do it.

You can stop deciding that you cannot stand this any more and start exploring how you *can* stand it. You can let go of who the person with Alzheimer's used to be and find out if there is anything in the here and now you actually enjoy about the changes you see—for example, perhaps he or she has become more accepting of affection and more relaxed about certain things. You can arrange a regular bodywork session for yourself to ease your tensions. You can talk to a counselor, therapist, or psychologist, or speak to your minister, rabbi, priest, or spiritual teacher. Call the nearest hot-line and complain anonymously if you wish. The list of what you can do to help your stress level is extensive indeed and has many different aspects from the physical to the emotional to the spiritual and psychological. It is limited only by your unwillingness to let go of your stress.

That may sound odd to you but, after all, only you can choose to deal with your stress. No one can take it away. You can ease it, if you choose to do so, or you can elect to stay addicted to it. There are caregivers whose relatives with Alzheimer's have been in full-time nursing home care for years who do not for one moment relinquish one iota of anxiety and frantic overinvolvement in the situation.

Yes, stress is addictive. It produces adrenaline, and we soon get used to the effects of adrenaline. We soon start to ensure that we are never without its jolting fuel injections into our nervous system. Many people are addicted to the high-energy tension of the adrenaline high. Researchers say that the adrenaline high is even more addictive than cigarettes, and this makes stress a hard habit to break. However, this habit is what burns out your system and brings about the physical and mental collapse that is not at all unusual among Alzheimer caregivers.

Ask yourself if you really want to let go of your stress. If your automatic reaction is "Yes, of course I do!" then ask yourself how you will let go of it. There are many ways, as you have just read. Look at your own reaction. Is it something like: "It's all very well for this author to talk, but I am much too busy, overwhelmed, and overworked to have the luxury of being able to do anything about my stress." The minute you find yourself with excuses for not letting go of stress, you know you are caught up and addicted. Look at your excuses—no time, too much to do, too many things to worry about.

No time to breathe? No time to stretch? No time to take a bath? These are the excuses of a person who does not want to let go of stress. That may seem ridiculous to you—of course you want to become unstressed, you protest, it is just that you dare not relax for a moment in case you can never get up and face things again.

Most support group facilitators report that when individuals and families are showing extreme stress—always busy, always anxious, always too much to do—it often seems that this stress is something they are holding on to to shield themselves from their own inner feelings.

Louise had attended a support group for seven years, starting when she had found out that her mother had Alzheimer's disease. Her mother never lived with her. She lived with her husband and, after his death, continued to live in the senior citizens' home they had chosen for retirement. As she become more ill, she was transferred into the full-care section of the home.

During all this, Louise never stopped dwelling on every negative aspect of her mother's illness. She was a constant source of negative stories and dire warnings to others who attended the support group. Her face grew more lined with anxiety, tension, and grief every month. Year after year, Louise poured out a stream of dark warnings and disastrous happenings. It was becoming increasingly clear to the support group facilitator that Louise actually hated her mother.

This was not surprising. By Louise's accounts, her mother had always been a spiteful and complaining individual whose dominating spirit had gradually stolen away her unmarried daughter's energy for life. Louise had partially covered up her feelings with a blanket of depression and anxiety, but it became obvious to most of the group members as time went by that Louise's problem was not her mother's Alzheimer's disease. Her problem was her unresolved negative feelings about her mother. When she fixated on the disease, she did not have to confront her feelings because she could blame everything on Alzheimer's. Eventually, Louise was gently guided from the support group into individual therapy.

Louise was an extreme example of a phenomenon often seen in Alzheimer care: the Overachieving Caregiver. It is this noble but embattled figure who is featured so widely in Alzheimer literature as a hero. It would be much more useful to suggest ways in which the OverAchieving Caregiver could let himself or herself (they come in both sexes) off the hook of being the best little caregiver in the world. It is not admirable to work oneself literally into the grave looking after someone else. It is a sign that a person cannot let go of control and has deep personal issues that need to be looked at.

Alzheimer's disease is hard enough to cope with. The caregiver does not need to carry this extra baggage that has become merged into the Alzheimer picture in our society. To learn to cope, it is essential that we deal with our own unhealthy patterns, not blame them on disease.

Every caregiver probably wants to do well by the person he or she is looking after. That is usually the essence of undertaking someone's care. So how do you know whether you are in danger of being an Overachieving Caregiver? Ask yourself the questions below.

Are you an Overachieving Caregiver?

1. Do you feel that no one else can look after your relative as well as you can?

2. Do you go for weeks without taking even an hour off?

3. Would you feel you had abandoned your relative if you took him or her to a day respite program?

4. Do you feel that only you can understand him or her and that letting others provide care would hurt, frighten, or otherwise damage your relative?

5. Do you feel anxious, exhausted, or irritable most of the time?

6. Do you secretly feel angry with your relative, and then feel deeply ashamed of your unnatural feelings and become obsessed by guilt?

7. Have you dropped all your previous hobbies, friends, and interests?

8. Would you rather die than let your relative go into full-time professional care?

9. Do you avoid going to support groups because you could never share your feelings with strangers, and/or you are sure such groups are full of people who just make each other miserable?

10. Do you keep all your fears, needs, and feelings to yourself because you aren't the kind of person who shares such things with others?

11. Are you sure that no good caregivers can be found?

More than two yeses qualifies you for the Overachieving Caregiver club. Welcome! There are many of you out there, and many of us who are involved in working with Alzheimer families would like to see this club closed down for lack of membership. Only you can decide to leave this particular club, however. You may still think, even after glancing down this list, that there must be some mistake. You are not an overachiever, you are just doing your best—and indeed you probably are. However, you could probably do far better if you would think about modifying your caregiving a little.

DO take your relative to day-care respite programs. He or she will probably enjoy it much more than you think. You are much too busy to provide the attention, fun, and activities that the program offers. Often people find it extremely comforting to be among others with the same level of ability. Of course, this means giving up a little control over your relative.

DO join a support group. They really do work for people. Most people who join them felt exactly as you do right now. It is scary to go to strangers and be prepared to share your struggles with them. It means you know in advance you can't control what will happen.

DO admit that you are not a perfect caregiver. That allows you to admit your anger and get it out of the way. It allows you to admit your impatience and stops it being your secret burden. It allows you to allow someone else into your little universe of caregiving. Of course, you won't always be able to control that someone else as tightly as you think you control youself.

DO stop trying to fool yourself that you are indispensable. You are not the only person who can meet the needs of the relative you look after. Actually, others may do some of it better than you do, so give them a chance to do it and let yourself off the hook a bit. That probably means letting go of trying to control yourself so much.

DO take a long hard look at your real feelings. You may be trying to stifle your emotions by concentrating solely on another person. You may well be sitting on a lot of fear and a lot of anger, old and new. Perhaps you resent your loss of freedom, or the ruined life you feel you have now compared with your dreams of golden years of retirement. Perhaps you even find yourself disliking your sick partner because of his or her constant needs. Maybe in your heart you think, "Yes, I did say for better or for worse but this wasn't included in worse when I said it."

These are the usual feelings human beings get uncomfortable about when caught up in long-term stress situations. None of us likes to get caught out in mean or spiteful feelings, but it is only a measure of the conflict that stress creates in us.

As you begin dealing with your stress, you will find that you become much freer to cope with things. You will discover interesting new solutions to old problems. You may well find an interesting new you that comes up with a whole new way to arrange life. If you make room in your life for yourself and for knowing your own needs, you will certainly find solutions that work for you.

CHAPTER 11

Knowing When to Let Go

....

*"I never wanted to put Christian into a nursing home.
I took care of him as long as I could. My daughters wanted
me to have him go somewhere but I wouldn't. Finally, I had
to. He got to be more than I could deal with. At night he
would get berserk and one time I had to call the police. I
couldn't handle him. My daughters said it would be best for
him. It was very hard to let him go."*

—EVELYN, age 84, whose husband died seven weeks
after going to a nursing home

It is often very hard to face putting someone you love into a
long-term care situation, knowing that you will never have
that person living at home with you again. Sometimes, however,
it is exactly the right thing to do. For other families, it is the last
thing they would ever do. This chapter will help you estimate
what is needed in your case and will suggest some possibilities
you may not have thought about.

If you are planning to keep someone at home, it is vitally
important you educate yourself about being a caregiver. Get to
know the disease and the task of looking after yourself too.

Thelma told her support group about her problems with
her husband Mel: "So I tell him to put his socks on, and do you
think he'll do it, the old devil? Not him. He just sits and glares at
me, all baleful like. And boy, you should see that man when I'm
trying to hurry him up for the doctor. He gets slower and slower
till I could just about brain him."

Thelma learned from other people in her group to change
her communication style—to cajole instead of order, to persuade

190

instead of demand. She also learned from her group that there were many ways of getting help. For example, Mary and Irving had a live-in student from China who earned board and lodging and a small salary in exchange for spending ten hours a week helping with Irving. Irving liked the young man and helped him learn English and Mary got extra free time for herself.

Live-in care can get as innovative as you want it to be. One lawyer decided to get help for her mother with Alzheimer's. Through her church, she found a newly arrived Laotian family who needed a home and work. They were a young couple and two children aged 8 and 10. They spoke little English but the lawyer's mother was losing her language skills. The family treated the mother with love and respect and looked after her well. She enjoyed being cared for by them and they had an easier entry into their American life. The arrangement was so successful that after three years, when the lawyer's mother died, the Laotian family stayed on in the house, now renting it. It was a successful experiment for all parties.

Being innovative can be the best way to deal with getting that extra help. The traditional pattern for hiring live-in help is to have one person for five days straight, then relief for two days. However, this care pattern is based upon the needs of the physically ill or frail elderly. It is the worst way to deal with Alzheimer care. It results in caregiver burnout and poor care, although it is an issue not being dealt with by caregivers, families, or care agencies.

Another innovative care situation was that of a 79-year-old woman being cared for by four live-in caregivers, all of whom received room and board and pocket money. They shared the caregiving schedule and led their own lives as well. Each of the four did caregiving one or two days a week and followed her own pattern, which created a much more interesting life for the woman they looked after. She did well with this arrangement. In a year she underwent no drop in functioning at all.

Most people think that in Alzheimer's care the choices are home or nursing home, but there are several possible choices in between those, some of which are actually more appropriate for the person with Alzheimer's disease. Given that nursing homes routinely charge more than $3,000 per month for what is often poor Alzheimer care, it is hard to see why two or three families do not get together and find a house in which the impaired family members can be looked after by live-in caregivers on a much more personal basis.

The main factors that lead relatives to think about nursing home placement are:

- illness or stress on the part of the main caregiver
- incontinence in the person with with Alzheimer's
- problem behaviors in the person with Alzheimer's, especially various forms of combativeness

Combativeness is not inevitable in Alzheimer's. It does happen to some people and might be caused by the effects of the disease on the brain. That has never been proven. What can often be seen are reactive angry responses arising from incidents that often could have been avoided by better handling on the part of caregivers. In the same way, neither is incontinence inevitable. Ninety percent of people with dementia are incontinent only if not reminded to go to the bathroom often enough. They have not lost control—they just forget.

Think about what would cause you to place the person you look after into full-time care. Think about your own health and what threatens that. Caregiver stress alone causes many placements, so take care of yourself. This disease does not necessarily require placement into full-time skilled nursing facilities. Apart from accidents and illness, the main reason for placement is that your family member needs more care than one person can give. Honestly examine the needs of your relative and, if they are more than you can give, it may be time to look at placement.

It is not always the deprivation you may think. For some people, their own home becomes irrelevant and even distressing. They do not recognize it. They are not really able to have their old life. Home does not feel homelike any more. They may do better in an environment designed especially for people who are impaired.

There, however, comes the rub. There are extremely few facilities where impaired people can really be at home. The hospital-patterned nursing home is often the least suitable environment of all. The hospital-like routine, the alienating clinical look of such places, the lifestyle based on nursing care—often irrelevant to the person with Alzheimer's disease—are destructive of the person. Even though such places claim to have day long activity programs, such claims can be spurious. Often only one or two staff members are available for activities with 50 or 60 severely impaired people.

Dementia-specific environments are now being developed that try to create homelike atmosphere with a protected ambiance. These give the residents the freedom to wander in safety, to interact with each other or not, and to be led into activities that enhance their lives. There are also many small care residences across the country. They are called adult foster homes in some states, home care residences in others.

If you are thinking about placement, which should you choose? How do you know what you should look for in a nursing home, a program, or a residence? The choice is hard, but the following guidelines are based upon years of looking at the good, the bad, and the ugly in full-care placement. Use them while doing your homework.

The first preparation comes from you, the caregiver. Finding the right place requires lots of homework. Avoid the crisis situation in which you overstress yourself looking after your relative and then make an overnight decision about placement. Look well before you need a place. Good homework takes time. That homework will repay you by enabling you to find a place where your relative can be happy and loved in good care.

In general, families tend to think that paying out large sums of money takes care of buying good care standards. This is totally untrue. High prices do not guarantee good care. Other things that do not guarantee good care are fancy wallpaper, well-written brochures, and staff members with nursing degrees. By now, you are probably wondering how you can find your way if none of these things helps you make a decision.

Start by examining the general category of care you want. So-called skilled nursing care does not mean anything in terms of Alzheimer-specific care. The phrase skilled nursing often refers to the kind of care a mother gives her baby, not to any high-tech training. Too many nursing homes are running

Alzheimer detention centers, geriatric prisons where sad inmates wander up and down the corridors all day.

Fortunately, many states now have more stringent regulations about how residents are to be treated, but there are many ways to pay attention to the letter and ignore the spirit of the law. A facility could pass an official inspection with no faults and still be a bad place for people with Alzheimer's to live in.

Unless the person with Alzheimer's has other medical conditions that demand nursing care or is actually bedridden or unable to walk unaided, consider a small home or adult foster care, if there is no really forward-looking Alzheimer-specific care residence in your area that you can afford. If you do need to choose a nursing home, find one that claims to offer special care of dementia patients, then visit it more than once. Be skeptical of any claims made about Alzheimer-specific care.

The reason for being skeptical is that hardly anyone yet knows what Alzheimer residents really need for their happiness and welfare. Most facilities are concerned about efficient containment of residents, and much less about their real well-being. Often, Alzheimer residents are seen as having less status and are treated as if they had indeed lost their minds. This can be subtle. Evidence of this downgrading might be that the Alzheimer unit is tucked away out of sight and its residents are not encouraged, even with relatives, to visit together in more open areas of the nursing home. Alzheimer residents often get less in the way of outdoor space than do other patients. Their recreation rooms may be smaller, or be used mainly for dining.

How can you tell whether the place you think looks good actually is good? Here are some ways to test it out.

Go there in the morning and notice how people are being treated. Is anyone being scolded for incontinence? Has someone been left half-naked in the corridor while waiting for a shower? Are the staff friendly or resentful? Can you smell urine? Go back at mealtime. Are people being treated with respect? If they need feeding, are they being fed considerately or is the staff member virtually force-feeding them without waiting for them to set their own pace? Notice in general the staff attitudes. Are they loving in voice and manner to residents? Do they actually listen to what residents have to say? Do they make fun of them? Are they ordering residents about as if they were children?

The other thing you will want to do is inquire about their Alzheimer-specific program. Too many nursing homes claim to have special care units for people with dementias when all they have is a set of doors with alarms. They actually offer nothing in the way of special programming for people with Alzheimer's. Ask to see the activity program schedule, which by law is supposed to be posted on the walls of the unit. Such a program should include art, music, socialization, exercise, and other specific activities such as sewing or crafts. A good program is based on here-and-now activities that are not memory- or cognitively-based. A good program also requires the participation and support of nursing staff. An Alzheimer unit that expects its activity staff alone to run the activity program is neglecting the well-being of residents. Any program it claims to be offering is spurious, since very impaired people often need one-on-one interaction at a low level of demand and response. You should be able to see some of these people getting such attention on your visits. Sit through some of the activities and ask yourself, would this add any pleasure to my life?

Often the alleged content of such a program is not as important as the actual quality of interaction being offered. People living in Alzheimer units are often very lonely, even though they are surrounded by others and get a lot of washing, dressing, and feeding attention from the staff. On the whole, few people listen to them. Fewer still take time to hold their hand or hug them. The more impaired people are, the lonelier they will be.

Therefore, what really makes a difference to them is whether anyone stops long enough to have even a tiny interaction. As an example, Agnes was a deeply impaired resident of an Alzheimer care unit. She could not walk, never spoke, and never joined in any activities. She had a look of great sadness on her face. Because she was so impaired, she tended to be neglected in all activities. She was wheeled into activities and then abandoned there in the middle of them. Often, because she never spoke, she was forgotten about and was left alone in a corridor or in the dining room.

A new staff member was struck by the sadness of Agnes's face and decided to try to work with her. For a few minutes several times a day, she sat with Agnes, sometimes held her hand gently, put a soft toy into her hand, or closed her hand around a foam-rubber ball. Agnes responded to this. Sometimes she would almost smile during these sessions. The staff member noticed that Agnes actually tried to roll the ball to another very impaired man, Walter, at the same table. Neither Agnes nor Walter could speak.

In the next few days, the staff member made sure that Agnes and Walter were put next to each other in their wheelchairs. One day, she found that Agnes was holding Walter's hand. There is no happy ending to this story, but there is a lesson. The lesson is that from such a tiny and, to the outward eye, unimportant activity, two extremely lonely human beings were able to have some real human contact in an otherwise ungiving environment. A good program would watch out for such residents and make sure they had the attention they needed. Many programs would continue to ignore them.

Beware of programs listing bingo, reality orientation, and reminiscence. These are largely irrelevant to people with Alzheimer's. Look for a place that has a healthy allowance for wandering, and make sure that any claims to allow such freedom are true. One nursing home made the claim that they had 10 lovely acres for residents to walk through in total safety, but they also had 33 out of 36 residents tied into wheelchairs. If there is no freedom to wander safely, forget that place. People with Alzheimer's often need to be able to walk as a stress leveler. Constant restrictions on walking cause high levels of stress. Is there a wandering path into a garden? That would be the ideal. The sad fact is that prisoners in San Quentin get a larger exercise yard than most residents in Alzheimer units in this country.

Look for a routine free of the unnecessary constraints of nursing-type schedules, which are for the convenience of staff, not residents.

Watch out for the following bad signs:

- A large percentage of residents tied into wheelchairs with back belt supports. This is the only restraint allowed by state law. It is supposed to prevent falls in those whose condition requires it. If a large number of people are tethered this way, it suggests illegal restraint of residents.

- A low activity staff-to-resident ratio. If you find 2 activity people to 50 residents, you can depend upon it that this nursing home does not have a suitable program for the demented. The ideal ratio would be one activity staff member to eight residents. Check out activities. Notice what goes on—is it appropriate? Is it demeaning? How many of the residents are really taking part? Are most of them just slumped in chairs? If a movie is shown, how many people are actually watching and noticeably enjoying it?

- Staff sitting or standing about talking to each other while residents sit slumped along corridors, ignored.

- Slow or no response if you point out that a resident needs something. "I'll tell her nurse," is a typical way to avoid meeting a resident's immediate need.

- Unattractive food.

- Bad smells.

- Residents improperly dressed, needing to be cleaned up, or without socks or shoes on.

- A high number of residents with bruised or otherwise injured faces, which indicates not brutality but falls. This could show lack of supervision or too much medication.

- No access to outdoors or no patios big enough to allow walking and a sense of freedom.

Hang around until you have seen enough to form an opinion. Talk to family members of residents and ask them what they think about the place. As well as your on-site research, check out the facility with the state licensing department. The department that licenses nursing homes (this varies from state to state; ask your local senior services agency) has to keep available for public reference their reports on every facility. These reports also contain complaints and follow-ups. Read recent reports. What violations have been noted and how significant do they seem to be? Are they noted as being rectified or do they recur?

This will give you one insight into that nursing home. You can get another by contacting the local Ombudsman office. The federal Ombudsman program which operates in every state, is a long-term care advocacy agency that oversees complaints about long-term care facilities—nursing homes, adult foster homes, units big and small. The Ombudsman volunteers go into facilities to investigate complaints. Local offices often have good insight into the underbelly of local care homes. They are likely to warn you about poor ones, and they are happy to tell you which ones rarely have complaints made about them.

All of this will give you a much better idea of what is out there. Do not let the lack of top-notch places depress you. The sad fact is that there are too few really good places, but you only need one. Do not be impressed by any amount of dressing-up done to the nursing home. One nursing home in the San Francisco area spent hundreds of thousands of dollars revamping the decor—into a slightly depressing light blue ambiance—and had nothing left over to buy a few benches so that Alzheimer residents could sit outside on the tiny patio that was all they had for exercise and fresh air.

For many families, it would be much healthier to choose a home care residence, a small homelike place probably with six or eight beds. Typical costs for these range from $600 (based on Medicare rates) to about $2,000 per month. Usually in such places people share bedrooms, but this is not necessarily a bad thing for people with Alzheimer's. They often feel frightened and lonely by themselves, since they tend to live in an unidentifiable timeless place, and having another person around can be comforting. This does not mean there will not be occasional quarrels, but they are not necessarily a bad sign either. People who share rooms are bound to raid each other's clothes and closets, but this is to be expected in Alzheimer's. It is possible to find care residences that offer individual rooms, but the rates are higher and it is not necessarily more pleasing to the residents.

Most people adapt surprisingly well to home care. It is small enough to preserve that feeling of normalcy, but is structured especially for a person who needs a lot of help with everyday living. Usually people in home care residences get help with whatever they need—washing, dressing, grooming, food preparation, and so on. They get what in nursing homes is often described as skilled nursing. Usually such places have alarms on the doors. Ideally they should have yards for residents to sit in or garden in.

You can check a home care residence out just as you would a nursing home. Visit and see what you think about it. Here are the warning signs to look for:

- Television on all the time, being used as an electronic babysitter.
- Radio on and tuned to a rock station. Even if caregivers try to find appropriate music for the residents, all too often they have no idea that popular music to their residents means 20s and 30s tunes—not 60s. Classical music or some soothing light background music is preferable.
- Bad smells.
- Improperly dressed residents, unless they have chosen this state of dress for themselves and are being respected for their choice.
- Cold, uncaring caregivers. Caregivers should be cheerful, upbeat, and obviously kind. Disgruntled, angry caregivers are probably overworked and underpaid. Some may also have alcohol or drug problems.
- No activities and no outings. There should be regular outings every week—to a senior lunch, to an ice cream parlor, to the park, to something somewhere. Ideally, there should also be activities in the house such as exercises or pet visits.

An ideal care home might have any or all of the following:

- A pleasant garden.
- Some pets.
- Planned schedule of activities.
- Good food.
- Regular staff training and little turnover of staff, although this can be an elusive goal in an industry where workers are often ill-paid. Staff should be responsive to your needs and those of your relative, not resentful of your expressing them.

The typical care home is a personal residence in which the home care part is paying for the real estate. Either the owner lives there or has a live-in manager, in which case the owner visits frequently. A good place has the owner on site most days, since home care staff need encouragement to keep standards high. In the last few years, the care home business has attracted many Asian-Americans, often those who are fairly new to this country. That is because it is an industry that anyone can enter; they can use natural human gifts for caring and in the process acquire real estate ownership. Some families worry because such owners do not necessarily speak English as well as they would like.

However, this is a situation that improves as people live here longer; moreover, good English is not nearly as important as a good heart. Many Asians tend to have an accepting and kindly attitude toward the elderly, which tends to overcome any small problems with language communication.

You may worry about whether choosing a home care residence will mean problems when, or if, your relative later needs the level of care offered in a nursing home. There is some trauma attached to any move for a person with Alzheimer's. A move will often bring about a temporary loss of functioning, which may slowly curve back upward but may never return to original levels. The choice must be a personal one. You may opt for a one-time-only choice and therefore go straight for the nursing home.

However, it is important not to undervalue the pleasure of life in the moment. However much you suffer to see your relative becoming more ill, it is likely that your relative can still experience a lot of happiness in the average day. The most supportive and friendly environment for the individual's functioning would always be a good direction to go in, even if it means a second move later on. It is a sad fact that people often die in the first few weeks after admission to a nursing home. Some of that mortality rate arguably has to do with the shock of entering an environment that does not really support individuality.

That move might never come about. For one thing, it may be possible for your relative to stay in the home care residence until death. Local authorities can be understanding of the need to keep someone in a familiar environment. Moreover, we can never predict how or when someone will die. You may worry at length about the classic Alzheimer death as you imagine it—bedridden, semicomatose, diapered, fetal—but it actually occurs quite rarely. In fact, most people with Alzheimer's die earlier of other things, including strokes, cancer, and all the usual suspects. So try not to make a decision now based on some imagined future. Rather, take the situation now and ask yourself where your relative would be the happiest. If you know of a good Alzheimer-specific residential program near you, by all means check it out. There will be more such programs as time goes by, and we must hope that they will offer the environment and care that a person with Alzheimer's really needs and seldom gets. What would that be? The ideal Alzheimer environment would include:

- a bright, cheerful building with lots of life-giving primary colors to offset the tendency to depression that is common in persons with Alzheimer's
- a homelike atmosphere with individually furnished bedrooms, ideally with home-like furniture
- wandering paths to lead the person along and back again to some central point
- safe access to outdoors and real freedom to wander at will in a protected environment
- high staff-to-resident ratio, with no cheating on the numbers. That ratio must mean staff who are actually available for relationship with the resident
- therapeutic programs through art, psychology, support groups, music
- lots of soft warm places, chairs, toys, blankets—all the things that give children comfort, because people with Alzheimer's allow their inner child to emerge quite often, or perhaps their child overwhelms them
- room for family members to stay and take part in programs, to spend time privately with the resident, and to undertake support group activity
- respect for the spirit and heart of the resident as shown by environment, treatment, and program elements
- gardening, indoor or out
- pet keeping

- therapeutic normal-life programming, such as helping out with carefully structured tasks, doing gardening, feeding birds, and so on

There are few programs like this, unfortunately, but we have to hope they will soon increase.

Making the actual transition may not be easy for you. You could take your relative along for a friendly visit to the place you have in mind and see how that goes. It may at least help put your mind at ease. If the visit goes well, you will probably feel better about allowing the placement. Of course, if you are already burnt-out as a caregiver, placement will probably come as a welcome relief to you. If you have close emotional attachment to your relative or spouse, you may feel sad and as if you are abandoning someone you love. You are certainly not abandoning that person—the bill alone, alas, will remind you of that—but you are buying care you cannot supply any more.

Expect to feel both relief and great sadness at first. There is no ideal way to decide how to proceed at placement. Some people go on a brief vacation for a few days, to get a much-needed break and to let the person settle in. Given that time is such a meaningless concept to the person with Alzheimer's disease, it probably does not make as much difference as you might imagine if you go away for a few days after placement. People with Alzheimer's notoriously do not have their time sense in place. The best thing, therefore, is to deal with your own greatest needs at placement.

If your greatest need is to go away and get some peace, do that. If your need is to see your relative every day, begin by doing that. Pay no attention to staff who tell you it is best for you not to visit your relative at first. There are no rules that apply to everyone. No one knows what the right thing for you and your relative will be, so do what you want to and take it from there.

Most people with Alzheimer's appear to settle into placement reasonably well. They tend to be cooperative and accept their new residence. Often they will become much more obviously demented. It is as if they have the freedom finally to give way to the true extent of their illness. There is no more need to cover up. Thus the new arrival often shows a downturn in functioning.

Do not let this worry you. It is the shock and trauma of environmental change. People recover from this, especially if the environment is supportive and they receive enough love and reassurance from staff.

You may find that your relative weeps when you visit or alternatively is angry or unpleasant, even though this behavior does not occur when you are not present. This is not a sign that your visit is disturbing or unwelcome. On the contrary, it shows that the person trusts you enough to let real feelings emerge. This will not always feel like a privilege, but it is.

You may not always find that things are as you would want them to be; no place is perfect. If you have been a really good caregiver, you may have to accept that no one will look after your relative as well as you did. You must adjust to the idea that good enough will have to do. Do not allow your sense of loss or grief or guilt to become inappropriate anger at the care facility. There will probably be a number of ways in which you find any place failing in the standards you would like it to have.

The biggest areas of complaint from families involve laundry, missing items of clothing, missing glasses and hearing aids, and other people taking the resident's belongings. Usually, the laundry is in some stage of processing, the clothes do indeed get passed around by the staff and the residents themselves, the residents do find all kinds of ingenious places to hide hearing aids, glasses, and teeth. All of this is normal. These are the most commonly heard complaints in both nursing facilities and care homes.

Actually, the most important real issues are food, kindness, and activities. If all of these are appropriate, you are already at an advantage. You may want to visit every day, but unless there is a real reason to do so, every two days is just as good. Even once a week on a regular basis is fine. You have to find your own balance between making a new life for yourself and nurturing your relationship with your relative.

If you have had to place a spouse in full-time care, you are almost like a widow or widower, even though you still have a living partner. You are not released from the burden and yet you do not get a real emotional reward. This is a very hard position, one often misunderstood by adult children. Many a spouse is expected to stay totally alone and lonely by children who do not in any way seek to fill the gap left by the placement of a partner. Go to support groups. Go to wherever you can to help rebuild your life. Treat yourself as if you were in part a widowed spouse, because effectively you are. Unfortunately, you might find you are not welcome in grief groups for actual widowed partners; such people may not, in their grief, understand your position.

You will need courage to explore your new life. Probably you will find mornings and early evenings the worst, so you should make a point of planning for those times. Go out for breakfast or early dinner or to see a movie. Take up visiting friends or family members at the hardest times. You will have to experiment to find out how to fill your life again. Take classes. Join clubs. And take what pleasure you can from being with your spouse on visits.

When you do go to see your relative, plan your visit. Take some items for mutual pleasure—food, photographs, music—or go for a walk or drive together. Take a photo album along sometimes so you can look through pictures together and go over memories. It might make you feel sad but it may also bring you both together again in those memories. Sadness will sometimes be what you feel. That's okay.

When you have completed your visit, do not make a special point of your farewell, particularly if your relative gets upset. You might just say, "I'll see you later, dear," and wander casually away. You might even warn a staff member you are leaving and do it without any notice. This may sound unkind, but it can often be less unkind than making a big deal of your departure if that causes distress. On the other hand, grief is natural, too. You will have to make up your own mind on this. Be guided by what you know of your family member.

Sometimes when you visit, you may feel that your family member is indifferent to your being there. Once people are in a full-time care residence that is now their life, it is very hard for them to make major adjustments back to the outer world. Transitions and changes are especially hard for people with dementia, and some people may simply make a decision not to deal with them or cannot deal with them. Therefore, they show no real signs of knowing their relatives, and make little effort to interact. It is easy for visitors to feel discouraged.

"She doesn't even know me—I don't know why I come," mourns Sam. He is right and wrong. Cognitively, his wife no longer relates to him as her husband. But she does sometimes address him as "Daddy" or as "Ronnie," the name of her long-dead brother. In using those names, she is stating, "I know you are important and close to me." Even when she does not show any signs that she knows Sam, staff members notice that she is calmer and happier when he has visited. Unfortunately, they have not told Sam this, so he does not know that his visiting changes his wife's emotional life.

Everyone who gets loving attention feels loved. That is the point of all visiting of the demented. As visitors, we may have to give up our desire to be recognized, acknowledged, and rewarded. We need to just be there for them. We go to see them not because they know us but because they are ours and they always need love. We recognize our connection and honor it. No matter how far they seem to travel away from us, out into that sometimes distant world of Alzheimer's, there is always a heart within them that is hungry for love and a spirit that responds to love.

Once we learn how to look for that—a certain expression in the eye, a touch from the hand, a slight movement of the mouth—then we will have it confirmed. Yes, the signs will say, I receive your love.

CHAPTER 12

Approaching Death

··

Death is often welcomed as the instrument of release for a
family living with Alzheimer's disease. In fact, the typical
Alzheimer's death usually comes gently, with the inward dreaming
of a person already absorbed in the internal process of dying, a
state resembling sleep or a turning away from consciousness. It is
nothing to fear. It has no pain or fearsome aspects. It is similar
to the way a child sleeps; gradually sleeps becomes deeper, consciousness weaker, until there is an end to life.

One of the most common questions asked by the families of
people with Alzheimer's is: What does a person with Alzheimer's
actually die of? It is a good question and, because of the nature of
Alzheimer's, one without a reliable answer. Although called a disease, it is more of a syndrome, a collection of symptoms gathered
in a body and a brain that is failing from the center, presumably
from the neurostructure of the brain itself. Therefore, when we
say a person has died of Alzheimer's disease, we are assuming the
death results from this failure of the system we label Alzheimer's.
Once someone has been diagnosed as having Alzheimer's disease,
that person's death, no matter what the actual cause, is likely to be
listed as caused by Alzheimer's. Similarly, people with AIDS are
listed as dying of AIDS when in fact they die of specific other
AIDS-related conditions.

Many people become obsessed by pictures of what they
imagine to be the real Alzheimer's death—the victim lying helpless in bed, being fed (perhaps intravenously), not speaking, not
moving, not responding, emaciated, needing to be diapered.
This is not at all the most usual fate of people with Alzheimer's.
On the contrary, it is quite unusual. Usually, people with

Alzheimer's die of the normal things we all die of—cancer, heart problems, lung problems, the many different ways in which we are ushered out of life.

Even in a special Alzheimer care unit, a 54-bed unit in a skilled nursing facility in the San Francisco Bay Area, only 2 out of the 54 people there were bedridden, even though many of the residents had been in care for several years. Of those who died in a three-month period, none died in a "classic" Alzheimer way. Five people died within weeks of admission to the unit, even though they had been in reasonably good health on their arrival. It is fair to assume that they died because of the trauma of being transplanted from a home environment into a sterile, clinical ambiance. Of the other deaths, one person died as a result of complications from falling, due to the side effects of psychotropic medications; two died of cancer; two had strokes and subsequently developed pneumonia; one had a cold that his family refused to have treated by antibiotics and he then developed pneumonia. This picture of the range of deaths is typical of Alzheimer's cases.

So, if you are facing the possibility of someone you know dying of Alzheimer's disease, do not envision dreadful pictures in advance. Actually, you cannot possibly know what that death will be like, so there is really no point in worrying about it until the time comes. In Alzheimer's, as in so many other difficult situations, taking life one day at a time is the key to managing stress.

There are some issues, however, you should think about long before you have to deal with them. The major ones involve making decisions about health care as death approaches. The most difficult issue for caregivers and family members is deciding what would be appropriate and acceptable medical intervention for the sick person. It is a good idea for everyone to make these decisions well in advance of need. All such issues should be decided upon before a time of crisis; few families can think completely rationally when face to face with an emergency.

Whether you decide to allow treatment of normally nondeadly conditions or not, you will have to think about the question of artificial feeding. Some people in the advanced stage of Alzheimer's disease are no longer able to eat. This is not the same as being unable to feed oneself or to chew whole foods, which are more common. Usually, these less serious problems are taken care of by adopting a liquid or pureed diet and having someone feed the person.

In some cases, however, towards the end of life, people become unable to take any food by mouth. This seems to be a failure of the body's whole system—cognitive, neuromuscular, and perhaps also emotional. It comes when life is effectively drawing to a close. Artificial intervention is often made at this point, either in the form of intravenous feeding or by surgically introducing a tube into the stomach.

This is a very personal issue over which people may deeply disagree. Even nursing staff can become emotional about this issue. One woman who wanted her mother to have a feeding tube withdrawn was shouted at by the director of nursing, "Do you really want your mother to starve to death?" Of course, she hardly felt that she could answer yes.

The main reason this becomes such a heated issue is that many people—medically qualified or not,—have never come to terms with death. Death is inevitable, for each and every one of us. After we are born, it is the only other thing guaranteed for any one of us. We may, heaven forbid, never make love, earn a living, or laugh, but we will die. Although we know technically we are not immortal, we generally live as if we are until life—and death—intervenes. When a person is diagnosed as having Alzheimer's disease, death is sending a message that it is on its way. Therefore, as a caregiver or concerned family member, you need to think through certain issues in acknowledgment of that message.

Most states now allow people to make major health care decisions and record them in some legal way. Some states, such as California, require families to record their wishes on paper when their relative is admitted to a care center. Since laws vary, you need to find out what your state requires for you to make your wishes known. It may only take a declaration to your doctor, but more likely you will need to sign a simple legally binding document. In some states you may have to get an attorney to draw up health care papers, either as a living will or as a power of attorney for health care. The power of attorney gives another person the power to make health care decisions on your behalf according to what is known of your wishes, should you become unable to indicate your own wishes in a medical situation. Everyone regardless of age or state of health, should do this. Anyone can have a serious car accident or a sudden disabling illness. If you have not done it before you reach middle age, you should certainly do it then, and you should make your wishes known to your family. Sometimes, medical decisions have been allowed on the basis of remarks made to family members, such as, "Mother always said she never wanted to be kept alive on a machine."

This commonsense matter is more complicated when a person has dementia. That is why all such health care decisions should be made when one is in the best of health. Once someone has been diagnosed with dementia, that person is no longer legally deemed to be responsible for making major health care decisions. There could be legal problems about any signed papers that are dated after the diagnosis of Alzheimer's. A court could argue that the person was not competent to make health care decisions. Such cases have been argued both ways in court. Many people with dementia and short-term memory loss can nevertheless have lucid moments in which they can indeed state their wishes clearly. A doctor or lawyer might well attest to that. However, if there was later a dispute about competency or about the motives of family members—for example, if the heir to a great fortune elected to switch off the parent's life support system—legal problems could arise.

In fact, most situations are straightforward and can be settled with little trouble. To avoid such problems, make health care decisions early. If they have to be made after diagnosis, consult a good family lawyer to have the relevant papers drawn up. You will often find that your family doctor is willing to co-sign health care papers, based on knowledge of the patient. In hospitals and institutions, usually the social worker will have all the relevant papers or will be able to help you assemble them.

All of this brings you face to face with the difficult question: How do you want your relative with Alzheimer's disease to die? When the course of the disease has eliminated the desire and ability to take nourishment, do you wish food to be forced? There are two possible approaches to the decision. One says that these people do not eat because they have a dementing illness that means they cannot make reasonable choices; therefore we should step in and get them to eat. The other says that after all, life does have a stop, and force-feeding someone beyond that person's ability to stay alive naturally is cruel and unusual; there comes a time to step aside and allow death to approach.

In the past—and it still happens—doctors intervened forcefully to insert stomach tubes, even against the wishes of relatives. In many cases, death followed soon after such intervention anyway, suggesting that the person was already dying before insertion. Then families were left with the decision about whether to have such tubes removed. One woman was in great distress about this.

"This is my sister-in-law and we love her dearly," the woman explains. "She's been bedridden now for two years and she hasn't eaten naturally for one year. They put a feeding tube into her stomach. Every night and every day for the past year, she has vomited and had diarrhea. We can't believe that she wants to stay alive like this."

The woman's dilemma was that she felt she and her husband were being asked to sentence his sister to death if they pushed for removal of the feeding tube. Actually, they should have been asked in the first place to make the decision about intervention. The dilemma they were faced with was a false one, created by what some people would regard as an unethical intervention by medical professionals.

Unfortunately, such situations still arise. Some states have made rulings that set precedents for intervention. Most opposition to moves to remove artificial feeding devices have come from nursing homes, perhaps because they feared being sued for allowing this. However, since they are also the establishments that directly profit from the prolongation of life under such circumstances, it is not easy to put their view forward as purely an ethical decision. There has to be a certain question of conflict of interest. A recent lawsuit in New York State established that nursing homes no longer have the right to force relatives to pay for care resulting from the artificial prolongation of life against their express wishes. This has undoubtedly changed a number of opinions about the process.

The way to take care of this issue is to make your decision long before need arises, and then find a nursing home or care facility that will honor your wishes. The most important thing you need to know is that people who have long been seriously impaired and are approaching death do not seem to experience any pain or emotional distress at the withdrawal of food. On the contrary, they seem to ease away into deeper and longer periods of sleep, often with times of some clarity.

One way to check this out is to ask the nursing staff of the hospital or care facility you are dealing with. They can probably tell you of some other patient currently in this position, and you could visit that person to observe for yourself. Become familiar with death. Be prepared to be around the dying instead of avoiding them. Only by getting to know the process will you feel confident about any decisions you make. You will find that normally when the time for dying is near, people naturally withdraw from the things that tie us to the world. Food is one of them. Toward the very end, liquids may be another. In spite of what you hear about people dying in two days with no water, people can go for a week or more without liquids in the dying process. People who are dying most often die peacefully and easily, especially if they are dying of the illnesses of old age.

It is ethically and morally correct to allow the dying to die. It may perhaps be unethical to try to drag them back no matter what. The biggest dilemmas come when someone has already been put onto life support systems. Then the family has to decide whether to turn them off. This approaches the issues of euthanasia, which has many ramifications for many people. This is why you should have your health care papers in place, so that unwanted interventions are not allowed to take place.

It is certainly dubious for medical practitioners who profit from such interventions to make the decisions. If you need help in making a decision, ask for assistance from the medical ethics committee of the facility or institution in which care is being given. More and more such committees exist today, simply because medical care now calls for extraordinary decisions. It is hard to decide not to do something that could be done, especially in a medical climate that values the conquest of disease above all else, including the pain and discomfort of the patients.

Be willing to trust your instincts. If you are sure what your relative's wishes would be, then respect that, no matter what someone else says to you. Many medical professionals have real problems accepting death, and they may project these problems on you. Do not accept their projections. Do what seems right to you. You will be the one living with that decision for the rest of your life. On the other hand, if you really feel strongly that life-prolonging measures should be taken, you must choose accordingly.

To help you make decisions, consider the following questions.

1. Will intervention cause extra suffering to your relative? Do not believe anyone who tells you that tubes are not uncomfortable. If you have ever had a catheter, a nose tube, or a stomach tube inserted, you know they are uncomfortable.
2. Will this intervention keep your relative more comfortable or will it merely extend life, regardless of discomfort?
3. Is life extension more important than allowing a peaceful death?
4. Are you making a decision based on what makes you comfortable or what will make your relative comfortable?
5. Are you afraid to think about death? If so, be suspicious of your own choice for life no matter what its condition.
6. Read about death and the dying process.

Some excellent books on the subject are available. You can also often find good workshops being offered locally. Ask your local hospice helpers or contact your local AIDS organization, since both work closely with the dying.

Let us assume that you have made all your medical decisions and that your relative is dying. If no food is being taken, you can reasonably assume that death will occur within two weeks, give or take a few days. What next? You may want to consider whether to bring your relative home for the last days. You could undoubtedly get a great deal of help from your local medical services—nursing assistance, home health aides, medical devices to make care easier, hospice workers—if you wanted to do this. It is not easy. It is hard work, even with all that help, but for some people it can be a wonderful time of closure.

It is not something you have to do. You must feel reasonably comfortable with the idea, but do not let anyone put you off if you really want to do it. Although people talk of the dying needing skilled nursing care, what they usually need is the kind of care you would give a baby. Of course, an adult is much larger than a baby, and that is the main source of problems.

If there are no extra medical problems such as open wounds, tubes, or seizures, a person dying of Alzheimer's disease needs to be kept clean, dry, watered, and warm. You will be able to learn everything you need to know in one day. This is not to push you into such a decision, but just to realistically let you know what is possible. Most people will tell you why it is impossible and you need to know that actually it is entirely possible.

There are some excellent practical books about looking after the dying. They are listed in the bibliography. Your library probably has them or can get them for you. Your local public health nurse can also help you learn what you need to know about looking after your relative.

Much of what you will need is the ability to be still with the person. Whether someone dies at home or in some kind of medical care situation, the essential need of the dying is the same, the most neglected need of all—the need to have company. Unfortunately, the dying get neglected. They get a lot done for them and sometimes a lot done to them, but they also get left alone a lot. It is typical in a care facility for the door of the room to be closed and the resident to be left alone except for an hourly check to see if the patient is dead yet. In hospitals, the dying tend to be regarded as medical failures and therefore sometimes are treated as somewhat unwelcome guests who have not behaved quite properly.

Since we will all die, that attitude seems harsh. It is only a reflection of our society's inability to deal with death. If you choose, you can make the journey to death a very special time in your relationship with the person who has Alzheimer's disease. To do so takes your patience and your presence. People who are dying, with Alzheimer's disease or not, are usually very absorbed in the inward process of their journey. It is common for them to slip in and out of sleep, even to appear to be in a coma.

It is guaranteed that the person will at some deep level know that you are there. It is easy to think that is not true, but we know from many accounts of people in comas who later recover that they have a deep awareness of everything going on around them. They may not be able to do more than twitch or slightly open their eyes, but that is the only way in which they can respond. Many an unconscious person has squeezed the hand that is squeezing theirs, so never feel that someone is beyond being reached. It simply is not true.

Not much is asked of you in activity with the dying. You need not do much. Just practice being. Do not get absorbed in doing things—that is just a way of avoiding being with the person. Hold a hand, stroke a brow, lean gently against the person so he or she can feel you there. If this is someone you have never been close enough to—perhaps a parent with whom you have had a difficult relationship—this is the time to work on anything you have left to say. Standing beside the gates of death, most of us can find it in us to forgive. It will certainly be worth it to try to find forgiveness in yourself.

Even if this person has been harsh or cruel or cold to you, as you watch that sleeping face, you might be able to see that this person is once more a child—helpless, unable to speak or move, just like the baby who came into the world so long ago. Perhaps you can see that the child did not get the love that was needed, because you know that love makes children into whole adults and the only thing that maims them is lack of love.

Perhaps you can begin to open your own heart, which might feel sad or painful, to do what that person could not—to allow love to flow. If you do love this person, it is much easier, of course. If there is little to forgive, then you can concentrate on offering all your feelings of love. Put them in the touch of your hand or the tone of your voice. Do whatever occurs to you—sing songs, talk, tell stories, weep, laugh. Sometimes just sit there and think of all the love that you want to send to this person. Draw on all the extra support you can think of—spiritual figures who inspire you, loving relatives who also care about this person, all the happy and grateful memories you may have.

Let the person know he or she is not alone, that love will go along to death and perhaps beyond. Doing this has nothing to do with religious beliefs. It is just giving the acknowledgment that we as human beings need love right up to the gates of death. We need to know we are loved. We deserved that at birth and in our lives and, if we did not always get it, at least we can give it to another person as death approaches.

Even if someone appears to be in a coma, assume that everything you say can be heard. Strangely enough, even if a person is normally deaf, you can still be heard. Say all the things you want to say. Especially, talk about love. One woman tells of speaking to her sister, severely ill with Alzheimer's disease for many years and unable to talk for the past two years.

"I love you, dear," said the woman, stroking her sister's hand.

"And...I...you," whispered the woman who had not spoken for two years.

So, make no assumptions about anyone's inability to hear or respond. Death brings such an urgency even into the life of a person with Alzheimer's that incredible things can happen. People speak who could not speak. People come back who have been absent for weeks, months, or years.

"He couldn't speak," said one man of his father, "but I could see him there in his eyes. He hadn't been there for so long but before he died, he was there. Of course I can't prove it, but I am as sure as a man could be that my dad came back to me before he died. It's made all the difference to me."

Being present at the dying time can indeed make all the difference. That is why this is such a special time. Even if you have never been present at a death before, there is no need to be afraid. Most deaths are very quiet. Most people have an easy death at the last, even if their illnesses have been hard. It seems that nature itself takes people in hand and brings peace and ease even to a body that has suffered until then. Some researchers claim that the brain releases special calming chemicals in the process of closing down. Whatever the reason, most deaths are peaceful. Most people look like themselves after death, except that they often look younger. The lines and tensions of the face smooth out. It is as if a light had gone out quietly. People do not usually look frightening at all after death.

This dying time can be useful as a process of reconciliation. This is the time to let go of anything unresolved and the time to give what this person needs—unconditional love and caring. One way in which some people have come to acceptance of Alzheimer's disease is to take the opportunity it gives to love the person.

Recalls one daughter, Kim, "Of course I wish my mother never got Alzheimer's disease. It wasn't easy to see her getting less and less able to cope, but we've always respected each other. And as she got more ill, she let us get nearer her and be more loving and more caring. And I see it as maybe the only way that we could have got so close to her. She had a hard life when she was young. When she was old, she became almost like a child again, and I felt as if we were able to give her what she'd never had before. That's how I made sense of it to myself. I'm not saying that makes it all okay, but it helps a bit."

That is partly what the dying process is about, not only about giving to the person who is dying but also working through life's story and making some sense of it for ourselves. Those who work hard to be with someone in this process come to peace and resolution much more easily. Alzheimer's disease is very hard on family relationships, and many people feel bitter and angry after the devastation of this disease. While that is understandable, it does no good. If you feel embittered or angry, the dying time is the time to confront all your feelings. In trying fully to be with the dying person, to give that person all you have to give in love and kindness, you will be benefited.

Many people have reported that this is so, but only those who have tried it can speak truthfully about it. Many other people who did not try it or who avoided being with their relative at death are left for years afterwards with feelings of bitterness, anger, and fear. It is as if the act of giving love so selflessly heals the person who gives it. Those who do not come to such resolution are often driven to try to find it with others. Alzheimer's care programs are full of volunteers with unresolved feelings about the disease still trying to resolve them.

Being present at someone's death reminds us, once again, that there is never a moment when love is irrelevant or unnecessary. It also helps us to feel less afraid of our own death to come and more able to live life more fully. Try to use this difficult time as fully and in as heartfelt a way as you can. It will all be returned to you in healing.

Moving On

··

Whether you have placed someone in full-time care, or whether the one you cared for has died, either event requires that you begin moving on. Each has its special difficulties, but either way you have to find ways to bring closure of what has gone before.

Closure does not mean never looking back or having no more feelings about what happened. It simply means becoming as emotionally balanced as possible so that you are not held back by the past in a way that prevents you creating a new present. Closure brings a sense of completion to the past so that you may find new life. Death and placement are different, but they evoke many similar feelings.

It is hard for a spouse to place a partner into full-time care. Even if the healthy spouse is relieved to see a partner in someone else's care—and such a feeling is entirely natural—nevertheless, there is likely to be a complexity of emotions involved. Placement leaves an emptiness in the life of the caregiver. Even though there were probably many times when he or she wished to be relieved of the daily burden before, when it actually comes about, the caregiver often feels quite at a loss. Alzheimer's creates its own schedule and pattern dominating home life. Its constant problems set a timetable that cannot be ignored. When the partner is no longer around, suddenly the freedom can echo emptily. It is hard to be free to do anything at all, for then you have to decide what that anything is actually to be. In this new emptiness can come depression and listlessness, an aimless restlessness that does not allow relaxation. Even if relief is the predominant feeling, there is likely to be a sense of purposelessness and loss in the partner. When the partner had been reluctant to put a spouse into care, of course these feelings of loss will be even greater. It is a little like being widowed and yet not being quite free to get on with the mourning.

So, if you have placed a partner into care, you can expect a complexity of feelings. Loss, grief, perhaps a sense of great guilt, relief, pleasure at the thought of being free to have a life of your own—probably all these emotions apply. The first few days after placement, you may just luxuriate in being free to sleep undisturbed, but it is likely that sadness will catch up with you at some point.

If you can leave home for a while, you might find a change of scene is just what you need. It will give you a chance to reexamine your life away from the suddenly empty house. While you are away, make plans. Write down the things you would like to do, the ways in which you plan to restructure your life. Don't sit at home with all the time you need but nothing to do with that time. Put yourself back at the center of your life.

Keep a journal to help you sort things out. You may experience wide shifts in mood and feelings at this time, and a journal will help you keep track of yourself. This is the time to grieve too. Do not be afraid or ashamed to cry, if that is how you feel. If you mainly feel relief, accept it. It is very hard to look after another person in the way you have. Of course you feel relief.

You might find it useful to continue going to support group, or to start if you have never gone before. The participants know what your task has been like and they can offer a lot of moral support. Do not be afraid that they will condemn you for placing your partner in care. Other Alzheimer caregivers, of all people, know how hard the task is and they will be facing the same choice at some point.

Make your own visiting schedule and see your partner as often or as little as you feel is right for both of you. When you get specially lonely, you might like to spend more time there. For all the loss of placement, you can still go and be with your partner for a while. You can walk somewhere beautiful or drink coffee together and hold hands.

Your biggest task is likely to be that of rebuilding your life. You will probably have to make real efforts to do so, since it is likely your social life became fractured during your caregiving years. You might start in the same ways other people are advised to meet people—go to classes and activities that interest you, go to social events and social centers and, of course, do not forget to invite people to your house.

If you have had years of living a full life with your partner, there is a huge hole in your life. It will be hard work to socialize, and sometimes you will feel more lonely with people than by yourself. This is normal. It is how everyone feels in a new social scene. Keep persevering. If your spouse was always the one who kept social life organized, you will have to make an effort to take over that role or you may lose your friends. Friendship does not just happen. Like any relationship, it needs careful nurturing. You may have lost, or never had, the touch.

Read what you can that will help you. Rebuild your interest in hobbies—reading, cooking, fishing—whatever you used to like. Find more interests. Make a list of things you always said you would do one day when you had time. This is the time. Everyone needs some unfulfilled dreams to keep working on.

If you used to go to church or temple years ago, try it again. If you stopped attending because of religious doubts or organizational inadequacies in your religious institution, it may have changed—or you may have. Remember there is a religious life, based on human institutions, and there is a spiritual life, based on your own inner being.

Go see your children and get to know them better. Without your partner, you are likely to find you have a different kind of relationship with your children.

Find something to do that involves helping other people and reaching out to others.

If it was your spouse who had Alzheimer's, you will probably face the dilemma of whether to seek romantic involvement with another person. This is equally true whether you have placed your partner in care or your spouse has died. It is a very personal issue, one each person has to work out independently. Many do work it out without much trauma. It takes time and it takes understanding from others and their respect for whatever your decisions are. There are many variations of dealing with this issue. Some people maintain a sexual partnership with their spouse, at least as long as feasible. The law, by the way, says you have the right to spend conjugal time with your spouse in privacy in a care home or facility. You can always bring your spouse home for visits, too. Do not let anyone try to make you feel ashamed that you would still like a sexual partnership. It is nobody's business but your own.

Some people choose to spend social time with others to take on a sexual involvement. Some people would like to have a sexual involvement but their children object. It is astonishing how many children turn into puritans where their parents' sexuality is concerned. This is an issue you will have to take your own stance on. Your choices are your own and you owe nothing to your children in this area. You may have to struggle for your sexual independence but stick with it. Do what you need to do and guard your rights and your privacy.

You may find yourself troubled by guilt if you have placed a partner in care. Almost every older person has some shadow of feeling about the notion of abandoning someone to the workhouse. However, workhouses did not cost $3,000 a month; when you put someone into full-time care, you are scarcely abandoning them. You need to work on those feelings through your rational mind and to accept that your partner needed more care than one person could possibly give.

It is normal to feel anger and resentment toward someone who is sick with any disease, let alone a disease that demands as much from a caregiver as Alzheimer's does. This anger does not come from our rational mind but from our emotional center that feels abandoned or used or just overwhelmed by this long ordeal. Because we know that the sick person has not deliberately become ill, we may feel guilty about our own anger. If you feel overwhelmed by such feelings, you might find it helpful to talk things over with a professional therapist, counselor, minister, priest, or rabbi, or a social worker.

When your partner has died, allow yourself to go through all the complexity of grieving. Many people feel the presence of the person who has died for at least three or four days after the death. There is nothing strange about this feeling. It has been noted in all cultures in all ages. You are not going crazy. Weep, talk, or be occupied doing things—these are your ways of coping.

You might feel you have failed your partner, that you should have done more. This too is normal and, interestingly, tends to be felt by people who actually did all there was to be done. You might want to talk about your partner, or to stay private and quiet. There are no rules for dealing with death.

There are many support groups for the bereaved. They can be a useful source of help as you go through the grieving process. Typically, spouses report that, contrary to what you might think, the loss is usually felt more after about six months have passed. By then, often you are no longer getting the regular support of friends and family and there is less opportunity to talk about your partner. Life has settled into what can sometimes be a bleakness, especially if you have not worked on rebuilding a life for yourself. Keep on working at that.

If you have lost a parent to Alzheimer's, you may have a more complex set of feelings. Most children fear that they too will get the same disease that their parent died of. Every little slip of memory causes a lurch of fear as they wonder if it is a sign of disease. Such fears are natural and complicate the grieving process.

There are two processes involved in the loss of a parent to Alzheimer's: coming to terms with the death and coming to terms with the disease. Both are necessary. The child who does not come to terms with Alzheimer's gets stuck in the past, often weighted down by bitterness, anger, and fear.

Often, the people who become involved in Alzheimer respite programs are those who have not yet resolved their issues around the loss of a parent to Alzheimer's. The hardest thing to do is to sit down with our source of pain and be with it until we understand it and can move on. If, however, you can face the process, then working with Alzheimer's can indeed be a wonderful source of healing. It is much easier to accept Alzheimer's in a stranger. Working with Alzheimer's is one way of coming to a peaceful resolution.

Using your experience to help others is a healthy way to process your own journey, as long as you also do the inner work of resolution that is needed for you to come to peace. If you work on improving both your inner and outer worlds, you will find some of the answers to questions that troubled you so much. The question that is most useful is not "Why me?" but "What can this journey teach me?"

There are no surefire ways to find peace and resolution. Each person must find his or her own path. Each path must include some way of coming to quietness, some ways of facing inner fears and pains, some form of finding a lasting sense of love and compassion within oneself from which one can reach out to others. If this book does anything to help you along that path, it has fulfilled its purpose.

Appendix A:
The 10 most common questions
asked about Alzheimer's

....

1. *Is this a new disease?*

No. It is first mentioned by description in 500 B.C. by a Greek philospher, but it was formally named Alzheimer's disease in 1910 after a German doctor Alois Alzheimer.

2. *Is Alzheimer's what they used to call senility?*

Yes, except that the term "senile dementia" includes other dementias of old age, too. The word senile actually comes from the Latin word meaning "sixtyish." Sixty was very old in Roman times, when the average age of death was in the 30s.

3. *Is it true only old people get it?*

No. The youngest person diagnosed was 27, but it is more commonly seen in people over 65.

4. *What causes Alzheimer's?*

We don't know yet. A vast amount of research is being conducted, but studies remain inconclusive.

5. *Is it found everywhere or just in this country?*

All over the world. Researchers have found it in China, India, the South Sea Islands, Japan, and Western Europe. It cuts across all socio-economic levels and across all races.

6. *Does everyone with Alzheimer's get angry?*

No. However, anger is one of the classic reactions to having a fatal illness, identified by Kubler-Ross. The other stages are denial, grief, and acceptance, all of which are also found in people with Alzheimer's.

A seldom-acknowledged fact is that most anger in people with Alzheimer's is *reactive,* not self-generated.

7. *Do all people with Alzheimer's run away from home and get lost?*

No.

8. *Is there a treatment or a cure for it?*

Not yet.

9. *If there is no treatment and no cure, why bother to get it diagnosed?*

First, because there is a 15 to 20 percent chance that what looks like Alzheimer's is actually a treatable or curable dementia due to specific causes. Second, because families need to learn how to cope with it.

10. *If it can't be treated or cured, what can we do to help someone who has it?*

We can learn how to relate to the person with Alzheimer's, and thereby avoid the crisis of love which is central to families who don't (or won't) learn this.

Appendix B: Resources

....

This section will offer a suggestion list of resources and will also serve as your personal reference list to keep you prepared for meeting your needs as a caregiver. In it, you may write down the telephone numbers and addresses that you need to keep handy. You might also like to photocopy this section in order to have a ready reference for anyone else who may serve as an additional caregiver.

ALZHEIMER'S ASSOCIATION

The major national resource available for the families of those with Alzheimer's disease is the Alzheimer's Association. This nonprofit organization raises funds for research into Alzheimer's disease and related dementias and offers informational support to caregivers, as well as offering free support groups for everyone dealing with Alzheimer's disease. These groups are available all over the country and there is sure to be one somewhere near you.

The national toll-free number is 1-800-621-0379 (if you are in Illinois, 1-800-572-6037). That gets you through to head-quarters in Chicago. Ask for your local contact and also for the free set of informational brochures that will introduce you to the basics of Alzheimer's disease. The line is open from 8 A.M. to 5:30 P.M. Monday to Friday, Central time. If you prefer to write, the address is Alzheimer's Association, 70 E. Lake Street, Chicago, IL 60601-5997.

To find your local Alzheimer's Association number through your telephone directory, look under "Alzheimer's," or check your local public library's reference section.

A local Alzheimer's support group will usually offer regular meetings (once a month or more frequently), contacts with other caregivers, a newsletter, local referrals, and information as gathered and experienced by caregivers. Groups vary in personality and style, so try more than one if the first does not work for you.

LOCAL RESOURCES

These are likely to include hospitals, home health departments, clinics, and senior services agencies.

Hospitals may offer free or very low-cost classes in caregiving, stress management, problem-solving, and so on. Most hospitals now have a commitment to education and have a community education department. Ask them to put you on their mailing list. Check whether they offer library or resource center facilities. Often, you can borrow books and videos free.

Hospitals have social workers who can often guide you in the right direction for the care you need. These valuable individuals are usually overworked and therefore your persistence pays. Often, community hospitals have home health departments that may be able to supply you with additional help—providing home health aides, therapists of various kinds, sometimes just time off. The home health department will also usually be able to check your eligibility for such help. The more medical conditions that affect the person you care for, the easier it will be to get assistance in your home.

Hospitals and home health departments often keep a list of local caregivers for hire. Ask for it.

Specialty clinics, if they exist, may offer some or all of the same services. Check under Alzheimer's in the phone book.

Senior centers vary greatly but can offer a wide range of services, activities, and outings, many of which are suitable for a person with Alzheimer's. As a caregiver, you can get access to low-cost legal aid and free help with medical forms and tax forms. You will also get more information about community resources.

The Area Agency on Aging is a federally funded national resource available in every state. The agency can give you access to a great deal of information and resources from which you may find specific answers to your questions or needs.

Senior services appear under various headings in different states. Try elder services, senior services, health and human services, senior and disabled services under your local state, county, and city headings in the phone book.

Again, social workers are often overloaded with cases, so be precise with your needs and questions. Write down your questions and write down their answers or suggestions. If you cannot get what you need, ask for another caseworker or another resource and be persistent.

PERSONAL RESOURCE DIRECTORY

Family doctor:
Name: Phone:

Alzheimer consultant:
Name: Phone:

Alzheimer respite program(s):
Name: Phone:
Address:

Hours and days of operation:

Caregiver: [In this section, make a list of the friends, acquaintances, and hired caregivers who can be available in an emergency. However little you think you would use them, list their numbers here. In an emergency, time is of the essence.]

Name: Phone:

Name: Phone:

Name: Phone:

Name: Phone:

Hospital:
Name:
Address: Phone:

Name:
Address: Phone:

Medical information package: Put together whatever would be needed for emergency admission—insurance cards, Medicare card, Social Security cards, and so on.

Long-term care residences: [visit these places and check them out thoroughly so you know you could rely upon them to care for your family member if an accident or illness befell you and temporary or permanent placement became necessary].

Small Home Care Residence (also called Adult Foster Home):
Name:
Address:

Phone: Contact person:

Senior Residence (assisted living):
Name:
Address:

Phone: Contact person:

Convalescent Hospital/Nursing Home:
Name:
Address:

Phone: Contact person:

Emergency Numbers:

Hotline/Helpline:

PERSONAL MEDICAL INFORMATION

In this section, list all the relevant medical information that will help you or another caregiver in looking after the person with Alzheimer's.

Medical conditions: (apart from dementia)

Medications:

1. Name: Dosage: Frequency:

2. Name: Dosage: Frequency:

3. Name: Dosage: Frequency:

4. Name: Dosage: Frequency:

5. Name: Dosage: Frequency:

6. Name: Dosage: Frequency:

Emergency procedure: (give instructions)

Dietary problems:

Alzheimer problems:

Problem: (brief description)

Onset: (time or trigger)

Interventions: (list everything that works)
[Deal with all behavioral problems in the same way, using a separate worksheet or journal to help you keep track and learn from past history. For example, a problem behavior might emerge after a family visit or after a particular occasion. Writing it down will help you identify what is going on.]

General interventions that work:
(e.g. going for a drive, or eating ice cream)

Appendix C: Agency on Aging

The federal agency on aging has state and local offices all over the United States, and these offices can be a very useful resource. They usually list every social agency and program for elders, as well as being the signpost to all other forms of help available for you locally. Call them!

ALABAMA
Commission on Aging
136 Catoma St., Second Floor
Montgomery, AL 36130
(205) 242-5743

ALASKA
Older Alaskans Commission
Department of
  Administration
Pouch C-Mail Station 0209
Juneau, AK 99811
(907) 465-3250

ARIZONA
Aging and Adult
  Administration
Department of
  Economic Security
1400 West Washington Street
Phoenix, AZ 85007
(602) 542-4446

ARKANSAS
Division of Aging
  and Adult Services
Department of Social and
  Rehabilitative Services
Donaghey Building, Suite
  1417
7th and Main Streets
Little Rock, AR 72201
(501) 682-2441

CALIFORNIA
Department of Aging
1600 K Street
Sacramento, CA 95814
(916) 322-5290

COLORADO
Aging and Adult Services
  Division
Department of Social Services
State Social Services Bldg.,
  10th Floor.
1575 Sherman Street
Denver, CO 80203
(303) 866-5905

CONNECTICUT
Department on Aging
175 Main Street
Hartford, CT 06106
(203) 566-3238

DELAWARE
Division on Aging
Department of Health and
  Social Services
1901 North DuPont Highway
New Castle, DE 19720
(302) 421-6791

DISTRICT OF COLUMBIA
D.C. Office on Aging
1424 K Street, NW, 2nd Floor
Washington, DC 20011
(202) 724-5622

FLORIDA
Program Office of Aging
  and Adult Services
Department of Health and
  Rehabilitation Services
1317 Winewood Blvd.
Tallahassee, FL 32301
(904) 488-8922

GEORGIA
Office of Aging
878 Peachtree Street, NE,
  Room 632
Atlanta, GA 30309
(404) 894-5333

HAWAII
Executive Office on Aging
Office of the Governor
335 Merchant Street,
  Room 241
Honolulu, HI 96813
(808) 548-2593

IDAHO
Office on Aging
Room 108-Statehouse
Boise, ID 83720
(208) 334-3833

ILLINOIS
Department on Aging
421 East Capitol Avenue
Springfield, IL 62701
(217) 785-2870

INDIANA
Department of Aging and
  Community Service
251 North Illinois Street
P.O. Box 7083
Indianapolis, IN 46207
(317) 232-7000

IOWA
Department of Elder Affairs
Suite 236, Jewett Building
914 Grand Avenue
Des Moines, IA 50319
(515) 281-5187

KANSAS
Department on Aging
915 S.W. Harrison
Topeka, KS 66612
(913) 296-4986

KENTUCKY
Division for Aging Services
Department of
  Human Resources
DHR Building-6th Floor
275 East Main Street
Frankfort, KY 40621
(502) 564-6930

LOUISIANA
Office of Elderly Affairs
P.O. Box 80374
Baton Rouge, LA 70898
(504) 925-1700

MAINE
Bureau of Maine's Elderly
Department of
  Human Services
State House-Station No. 11
Augusta, ME 04333
(207) 289-2561

MARYLAND
Office on Aging
State Office Building
301 West Preston Street,
  Room 1004
Baltimore, MD 21201
(301) 225-1106

MASSACHUSETTS
Executive Office of
  Elder Affairs
38 Chauncy Street
Boston, MA 02111
(617) 727-7750

MICHIGAN
Office of Services to the Aging
P.O. Box 30026
Lansing, MI 48909
(517) 373-8230

MINNESOTA
Board on Aging
Human Services Bldg.
444 Lafayette Blvd.
St. Paul, MN 55155
(612) 296-2544

MISSISSIPPI
Council on Aging
301 West Pearl Street
Jackson, MS 39203
(601) 949-2013

MISSOURI
Division on Aging
Department of Social Services
P.O. Box 1337
Jefferson City, MO 65102
(314) 751-3082

MONTANA
Family Services Division
P.O. Box 8005
Helena, MT 59601
(406) 444-5900

NEBRASKA
Department on Aging
P.O. Box 95044
301 Centennial Mall South
Lincoln, NE 68509
(402) 471-2306

NEVADA
Division on Aging
Department of
  Human Resources
505 East King Street
Kinkead Building, Room 101
Carson City, NV 89710
(702) 885-4210
(800) 992-0900 (NV)

NEW HAMPSHIRE
Division of Elderly
  & Adult Services
6 Hazen Drive
Concord, NH 03301
(603) 271-4680

NEW JERSEY
Division on Aging
Department of
  Community Affairs
C N 807
Trenton, NJ 08625
(609) 292-4833

NEW MEXICO
State Agency on Aging
224 East Palace Avenue,
  4th Floor
La Villa Rivera Building
Santa Fe, NM 87501
(505) 827-7640

NEW YORK
Office for the Aging
New York State
  Executive Department
Empire State Plaza,
  Agency Building No. 2
Albany, NY 12223
(518) 474-4425
(800) 342-9871 (NY)

NORTH CAROLINA
Division on Aging
1985 Umpstead Drive,
  Kirby Building
Raleigh, NC 27603
(919) 733-3983

NORTH DAKOTA
Aging Services
Department of
  Human Services
State Capitol Building
Bismarck, ND 58505
(701) 224-2577

OHIO
Department on Aging
50 West Broad Street,
  9th Floor
Columbus, OH 43266
(614) 466-5500

OKLAHOMA
Special Unit on Aging
Department of
  Human Services
P.O. Box 253532
Oklahoma City, OK 73125
(405) 521-2327

OREGON
Senior Services Division
313 Public Service Building
Salem, OR 97310
(503) 378-4728
(800) 232-3020 (OR)

PENNSYLVANIA
Department of Aging
231 State Street
Harrisburg, PA 17101
(717) 783-1550

RHODE ISLAND
Department of Elderly Affairs
79 Washington Street
Providence, RI 02903
(401) 277-2858

SOUTH CAROLINA
Commission on Aging
915 Main Street
Columbia, SC 29201
(803) 783-3203

SOUTH DAKOTA
Office of Adult Services
 and Aging
700 Governor's Drive
Kneip Building
Pierre, SD 57501
(605) 773-3656

TENNESSEE
Commission on Aging
706 Church Street, Suite 201
Nashville, TN 37219
(615) 741-2056

TEXAS
Department on Aging
P.O. Box 12786
 Capitol Station
1949 IH 35
South Austin, TX 78741
(512) 444-2727
(800) 252-9240 (TX)

UTAH
Division of Aging
 and Adult Services
Department of Social Services
Social Services Bldg.
120 North, 200 West
Salt Lake City, UT 84145
(801) 538-3910

VERMONT
Office on Aging
103 South Main Street
Waterbury, VT 05676
(802) 241-2400

VIRGINIA
Department on Aging
700 Franklin Street
Richmond, VA 23219
(804) 225-2271

WASHINGTON
Aging and Adult Services
 Administration
Department of Social and
 Health Services
OB-44A
Olympia, WA 98504
(206) 586-3768

WEST VIRGINIA
Commission on Aging
Holly Grove—State Capitol
Charleston, WV 25305
(304) 348-3317
(800) 642-3671 (WV)

WISCONSIN
Bureau of Aging
Division of
   Community Services
P.O. Box 7851
Madison, WI 53702
(608) 266-2536

WYOMING
Commission on Aging
Hathaway Building-Room 139
Cheyenne, WY 82002
(307) 777-7986

Bibliography

....

This bibliography only features books that are actively helpful, supportive, and understanding of the caregiver and the person with Alzheimer's disease.

ALZHEIMER'S DISEASE

Alzheimer's Association: Brochures on a wide variety of topics involving Alzheimer's and caregiving, available free from the national headquarters in Chicago or from your local Alzheimer Association office (see Appendix for phone number and address)

L. Gwyther: *Care of Alzheimer Patients.* American Health Care Association and the Alzheimer Association, 1985. This book is one of the best available for general understanding of Alzheimer's disease. Even though it is aimed at nursing staff, it is readable, comprehensible and humane.

N.L. Mace and P.V. Rabins: *The 36 Hour Day.* Johns Hopkins University Press, 1981. One of the first guides to living with Alzheimer's. A comprehensive book covering all the issues. Slightly disorganized, but the first classic in the field.

F. Safford: *Caring for the Mentally Impaired Elderly.* Henry Holt, 1986. Despite its clinical sounding title, this is an excellent self-help book to get you through the everyday caregiving tasks. Good information on nursing and physical care and compassionate in attitude.

CAREGIVING

R. Dass and P. Gorman: *How Can I Help?.* Knopf, 1986. An excellent and wide-ranging book on the human issues of caring for others and finding the deeper sense of purpose within the task.

E. Kubler-Ross: *On Death and Dying.* Macmillan, 1969. A warm, human book on the issues of death and dying, practical and profound at the same time.

Red Cross: *Home Nursing.* This is out of print but you may be able to find a copy at a garage sale or in a secondhand bookstore. A practical handbook for the home caregiver that is still excellent and unpretentious.

GENERAL RESOURCES

Biracree, T. & N.: *Over Fifty: The Resource Book for the Better Half of Your Life.* Harper, 1991. This is exactly what it says, an excellent collection of resources for every situation affecting people over fifty. Easy to use, accessible, and very comprehensible.

UNDERSTANDING AFFLICTION

C. Brown: *My Left Foot.* An inspiring autobiography written (with his left foot) by a young Irishman born paralyzed and speechless due to cerebral palsy. This was made into an Oscar-winning film, which is available on video.

S. Luria: *Man With A Shattered World.* A fascinating and humane study of a Russian soldier wounded in battle who returned home with a head wound that affected his memory. The author is a famous Russian neurologist.

O. Sacks: *The Man Who Mistook His Wife for a Hat.* An entertaining book of neurological anecdotes that help us comprehend what it is like to live with an afflicted brain.

SPIRITUALITY AND CAREGIVING

H. Kushner: *When Bad Things Happen to Good People.* Schocken Books, 1981. Explores the overwhelming question "Why Me?" and finds some answers.

Mother Theresa: *Life in the Spirit.* Harper, 1982. A simple guide offering spiritual consolation in caregiving.

Rinpoche Sogyal: *Tibetan Book of Living and Dying.* Harper, 1993. A profound, yet practical, spiritual guide to working with the dying that can be used by caregivers of any faith or none.

Thich Nhat Hanh: *Being Peace.* Parallax Press, 1987. This unpretentious, powerfully simple book can help caregivers of all beliefs or none to find inner peace in everyday life and actions.

Index